THE WISDOM
of
DR DAVID R. HAWKINS

ALSO BY DR DAVID R. HAWKINS

BOOKS

*Book of Slides: The Complete Collection
Presented at the 2002–2011 Lectures with Clarifications*

Discovery of the Presence of God: Devotional Nonduality

*The Ego Is Not the Real You:
Wisdom to Transcend the Mind and Realize the Self*

The Eye of the I: From Which Nothing Is Hidden

Healing and Recovery

I: Reality and Subjectivity

Letting Go: The Pathway of Surrender

*The Map of Consciousness Explained: A Proven Energy Scale to Actualize Your
Ultimate Potential*

Power vs. Force: The Hidden Determinants of Human Behavior

Reality, Spirituality and Modern Man

*Success Is for You: Using Heart-Centered Principles for Lasting Abundance
and Fulfillment*

Transcending the Levels of Consciousness: The Stairway to Enlightenment

Truth vs. Falsehood: How to Tell the Difference

AUDIO PROGRAMMES

How to Surrender to God

Live Life as a Prayer

The Map of Consciousness Explained

Please visit:

Hay House UK: www.hayhouse.co.uk
Hay House USA: www.hayhouse.com®
Hay House Australia: www.hayhouse.com.au
Hay House India: www.hayhouse.co.in

• • •

THE WISDOM
of
DR DAVID R. HAWKINS

Classic Teachings on
Spiritual Truth and Enlightenment

HAY HOUSE

Carlsbad, California • New York City
London • Sydney • New Delhi

Published in the United Kingdom by:
Hay House UK Ltd, The Sixth Floor, Watson House,
54 Baker Street, London W1U 7BU
Tel: +44 (0)20 3927 7290; Fax: +44 (0)20 3927 7291; www.hayhouse.co.uk

Published in the United States of America by:
Hay House Inc., PO Box 5100, Carlsbad, CA 92018-5100
Tel: (1) 760 431 7695 or (800) 654 5126
Fax: (1) 760 431 6948 or (800) 650 5115; www.hayhouse.com

Published in Australia by:
Hay House Australia Ltd, 18/36 Ralph St, Alexandria NSW 2015
Tel: (61) 2 9669 4299; Fax: (61) 2 9669 4144; www.hayhouse.com.au

Published in India by:
Hay House Publishers India, Muskaan Complex, Plot No.3, B-2,
Vasant Kunj, New Delhi 110 070
Tel: (91) 11 4176 1620; Fax: (91) 11 4176 1630; www.hayhouse.co.in

Cover design: Julie Davison
Interior design: Bryn Starr Best

Excerpts from *Healing and Recovery* (2009) are used with permission from the author and publisher.

An excerpt from *Discovery of the Presence of God: Devotional Nonduality* (2007), Chapter 7: The Razor's Edge, p133 is used with permission from the author and publisher.

Excerpts from *The Map of Consciousness Explained: A Proven Energy Scale to Actualize Your Ultimate Potential* (2020), Preface, pxiv–xv, are used with permission from the author and publisher.

A catalogue record for this book is available from the British Library.

Tradepaper ISBN: 978-1-78817-683-5
E-book ISBN: 978-1-4019-6505-1

Printed and bound by CPI Group (UK) Ltd, Croydon, CR0 4YY

CONTENTS

FOREWORD

David R. Hawkins, M.D., Ph.D., affectionately called "Doc" by his spiritual students, died peacefully at his home in Sedona, Arizona, on September 19, 2012, at the age of 85. Even up to the last breath, he gave his all to help others. He left a body of work that includes over 15 books and hundreds of hours of audio-visual programs.

Those of us who had the great fortune to hear Dr. Hawkins speak in person will never forget what it was like. People from all walks of life, even from faraway countries, attended the sold-out monthly seminars he offered. We heard the material he presented, yet we experienced something deeper than words. The information was delivered via a carrier wave of Love, silent and all-pervading. Historically, this nonverbal transmission has been called the "Grace of the Teacher." Through his oral teachings, he conveyed profound truths in a personable way that awakened the inner Self of the listener.

A transformative effect occurs also through his writing. The late spiritual and self-help author, Wayne Dyer, called Dr. Hawkins's book *Power vs. Force* "perhaps the most important and significant book I've read in the past 10 years." Saint Mother Teresa of Calcutta wrote this to him after reading his manuscript for *Power vs. Force*: "Continue to use your beautiful gift of writing to the full." Legendary musician Nipsey Hussle, shortly before his untimely death, said to an interviewer: "The most powerful book I've read in the last ten years is called *Power vs. Force*."

Power vs. Force, Dr. Hawkins's first spiritual book, has sold more than a million copies and has been translated into more than 25 languages. He had wanted to publish it anonymously, for he said it came "through" him rather than "from" him. Of its significance, he observed: "The karma of mankind changed with the writing of that book."

That book was followed by *Eye of the I: From Which Nothing Is Hidden* and *I: Reality and Subjectivity.* These three books, he said, are the foundational "trilogy" of his teachings. From there, he wrote many more books to apply his teachings to all areas of life, from physical healing to overcoming addiction, to success and happiness. In 2019, a primer of his work, *The Map of Consciousness Explained,* was published to illumine the many facets of his key discovery, The Map of Consciousness®.

Surprisingly, Dr. Hawkins did not begin his spiritual writing until he was 65. This in itself is an encouragement to us, the readers, to trust his teaching that our lives contain hidden potentials waiting to be actualized when the time is right. In fact, the book you hold in your hand may be the catalyst needed to actualize a potential within you. He explains:

> That is the value of the presence of a Teacher whose energy field is like a catalyst. The high energy field of the Self is already present in the student. It does not have to be acquired but only activated, which is a consequence of positive karmic potentiality. — *Discovery of the Presence of God: Devotional Nonduality* (2007), Chapter 7: The Razor's Edge, p. 133.

This book is a unique and wonderful resource of teachings from Dr. Hawkins. It has been adapted from one of Dr. Hawkins's classic audio programs, and it gives readers the ambience of his oral conveyance. You might imagine that you are sitting there in his audience—listening and watching, laughing and receiving.

His wife, Susan Hawkins, who was always on stage with him as his lovemate, co-researcher, and "right arm," gave this account of his lectures:

When I was on stage with him, I saw how he would say things in a powerful way and suddenly people's faces would light up—they got it! It was so fulfilling to see that response and to know that someone's life was changed. For Dave, it was never about himself—he cared only about the message and its impact on others. He had a contagious sense of humor; it was impossible not to laugh whenever he was laughing. He didn't care about appearances or getting approval from others, because he knew who and what he was. — *The Map of Consciousness Explained: A Proven Energy Scale to Actualize Your Ultimate Potential* (2020), Preface, p. xiv.

As you read this book, you will perhaps realize why someone described his lecture style as a mixture of Einstein, the Buddha, and Mr. Magoo. He was a liberated being—free, spontaneous, compassionate, humorous, and totally available. His spaciousness welcomed everyone and everything. Being in his presence, you knew he saw into you, he saw through your facades, and he loved you exactly as you were. He addressed himself to the greater Self within you.

Though he appeared in the form of a man, he was somehow beyond male and female, human and nonhuman. He knew the Divine Light in all things; he recognized the sacredness even in the little beetle and the mother skunk. He *was* the "Eye of the I" from which nothing was hidden. Nothing existed that was not included in this Love.

He inhabited the rarefied realm of what the world calls "enlightenment," yet he was dedicated to helping others overcome the painful obstacles in everyday life. He strove to be helpful and ordinary. As you go through this book, you will encounter very advanced teachings coming through in the simplest way possible. The purity of the message is due to his total surrender of personal gain. There were no marketing schemes to make money. There were no robes or rituals, saintly affects or special incantations. There were no theatrics or miracles performed on stage. The true teacher, he said, has no interest in special clothing, dramatic performances, names or titles, for there is actually no "person" left who would care about such things.

As you will learn in this book, the trademark of Dr. Hawkins's research is his pioneering, internationally known Map of Consciousness. It incorporates findings from quantum physics and nonlinear dynamics, thereby confirming the classical stages of spiritual evolution found in the world's sacred literature as actual attractor fields. These spiritual levels have been delineated by saints, sages, and mystics, yet there had never been a scientific framework by which to understand the inner terrain.

The Map of Consciousness is clinically sophisticated in its depiction of each level's emotional tone, view of God, and view of life. For example, Fear views God as punitive, whereas Love views God as loving. The Map of Consciousness illumines heretofore unknown aspects of consciousness. With each progressive rise in the level of consciousness, the frequency or vibration of energy increases. Thus, higher consciousness radiates a beneficial and healing effect on the world, verifiable in the human muscle response, which stays strong in the presence of Love and Truth. In contrast, negative energy fields that calibrate below the level of integrity induce a weak muscle response. This stunning discovery of the difference between power and force has influenced numerous fields of human endeavor, business, advertising, education, psychology, medicine, law, and international relations.

Susan Hawkins explains:

Nearly every day, I hear from someone who says that Dave's Map of Consciousness changed their life. Some people have gotten free from heroin, alcoholism, and other hopeless addictions. Others have healed from various illnesses and emotional struggles. Whatever the life problem, the Map gives them the way out of their suffering. — *The Map of Consciousness Explained: A Proven Energy Scale to Actualize Your Ultimate Potential* (2020), Preface, p. xv.

Throughout this book, you will come to understand why the most important spiritual goal is to raise your level of consciousness. For example, Dr. Hawkins explains that the positive levels on the Map are correlated with greater immunity to disease, higher rates of happiness, higher job satisfaction, and overall greater fulfillment in life.

If these personal benefits are not motivating enough, he also explains that by raising our level of consciousness, we benefit all of life. Even a single forgiveness or a single act of kindness blesses everyone and everything. As we surrender our small self, the intrinsic life energy of the Higher Self is free to flow through us. As he says in this book: "The inner worth of every human being is infinite. Its potential is infinite."

Therefore, a prayer for readers of this book is to *become* that innate inner potential which is *infinite*. As Doc liked to say: "Straight and narrow is the way. Waste no time!"

—Fran Grace, Ph.D.

INTRODUCTION

Nearly 10 years ago, Dr. David R. Hawkins, M.D., Ph.D., died peacefully at his home in Sedona, Arizona, and his profound message of spiritual truth, enlightenment, and growth lives on to this day.

In this book, you'll explore the most classic teachings from Dr. Hawkins. In the following 10 chapters, his most important spiritual themes are covered, amounting to an unforgettable and life-changing experience.

A nationally renowned psychiatrist, physician, researcher, spiritual teacher, and lecturer, Dr. Hawkins was the founding director of the Institute for Spiritual Research Incorporated and the founder of the path of devotional non-duality. He lectured widely at such places as Westminster Abbey, Oxford Forum, the University of Notre Dame, the University of Michigan, and Harvard University. In addition, he was an advisor to Catholic, Protestant, and Buddhist monasteries. He conferred with foreign governments on international diplomacy and was instrumental in resolving longstanding conflicts that were major threats to world peace. He was featured in documentary films, magazines, and radio interviews, such as Oprah Radio and the Institute of Noetic Sciences, for his work in the areas of health, healing, recovery, spirituality and modern life, meditation, and consciousness calibration. You'll learn more about the specifics of the calibration process and the Map of Consciousness® in Chapter 2 of this book. However, Dr. Hawkins will refer to calibration levels (such as a calibration level of 190 or a calibration level of 210) throughout the book, so it can be helpful to have the Map handy as you read. The Map of Consciousness can be found online at https://veritaspub. com/map-of-consciousness.

At the end of this book, you will find a bonus chapter taken from one of Dr. Hawkins's lectures, "The Most Valuable Qualities for a Spiritual Seeker," in which he outlines the simple and powerful qualities that every spiritual seeker will need on the path to Enlightenment. This is one of the last lectures Dr. Hawkins delivered during his earthly journey.

Are you ready? Let's get started.

Chapter 1

MOVING FROM THE EGO TO SERVICE

The vast majority of self-help teachers encourage people to follow outward, assertive, ego-oriented methods to achieve long-lasting wealth and happiness. But, having traveled that path himself early in his life, Dr. Hawkins knew that the ego path was ultimately a dead end.

In this section, Dr. Hawkins will encourage you to step off the ego path onto a more rewarding, fulfilling, and service-oriented enlightenment path. And as he explains, the path you will travel begins with your personal choice.

Everybody's aware when they are faced with a choice between the high road and the low road. That's a common experience. For example, you could get a better grade by cheating or you could get an *honest* grade by not cheating. We have to make those decisions over and over.

To me, the dilemma of human existence is that you have to choose *every second*. Every second of every minute your mind is constantly making choices. The challenge of human existence is phenomenal when you look at it. But because you're used to it, you don't realize that.

Every single moment, when I speak, my mind is choosing words—how do I enunciate that word, how do I phrase my messages, contextualize them, amplify them. I'm deciding whether to explain myself more, or if I should just let the other person worry about it. So for every single word I'm choosing, there are probably 50 different possible options. I could suddenly become comical and break the seriousness. And for some people, that would help them; other people would say, "Oh, I can't believe what he's saying—he's just being lighthearted about things." They don't see the spiritual value of humor.

So the human, at every instant, every fractional instant, is choosing between this thought and that thought, between this option and that option. *Shall I shift in my chair?* I just had to decide that; there are probably half a dozen conscious options, and there's probably dozens of *unconscious* options, ways that we could go. *Should I encourage them to go in that direction, or should I discourage them from following that track?* We're always trying to influence, and we're always making choices. I always feel sorry for the human condition, in that you can never be content because the minute you're content, you're even wondering if you *should* be content.

There's very little rest for humans, because our minds are constantly presenting an endless array of options. People say they don't believe in karma. Well, you don't have to use that word. What you can see is that your mind is endlessly, constantly confronted with options, and your whole life is going to change depending on which option you pick. It's like a giant map, an electronic map, and if you choose this direction, you're going to end up hundreds of miles from if you'd chosen that other direction. So making choices is the major human occupation. Yet nobody ever mentions it. The major human preoccupation, and it eclipses all others, is the constant making of choices. *Should I look in that direction or not? Should I try to get this job? Should I say this or say that? Should I wear this? Should I walk on the other side of the sidewalk? Should I call so-and-so? Should I let this bill wait another two weeks?*

• • •

What you see is a projection of your own consciousness. It's what you project out into the world, whether you see this world as sad, happy, ludicrous, beneficial, beautiful, divine, frustrating, corrupt, evil, or an infinite good. If man is to progress to realize the ultimate divinity, which is the core of his existence, then it would require progressively growing into that dimension of awareness. The karmic benefit of human lifetime, as the Buddha said, would be self-rewarding. Fortunate it is to be born a human, even more fortunate it is to have heard of enlightenment; and rarer still is it to be born, to have heard of enlightenment, and then proceed to pursue it. And I might add, rarer than that is to achieve enlightenment, because it requires tenacity. The roadway to enlightenment takes you through difficult terrain, like a walk through a swamp.

Fortunate it is to be born a human, even more fortunate it is to have heard of enlightenment; and rarer still is it to be born, to have heard of enlightenment, and then proceed to pursue it.

THE DIFFERENCE BETWEEN FORCE AND POWER

Force is linear. Force is demarcated. It has a form like a molecule. It may have ears on it, eyes, feet, anything. It has structure. Therefore, force is limited. That which has form is obviously limited. It's limited by form. That which is formless is unlimited. Eventually, we can solve every riddle that's ever plagued mankind with this little simple formula.

We know that $E=mc^2$. This is force limited to form. Power, which is nondual, is infinite. Power has no limitation. In fact, the greater the demand you put on power, the greater it swells and meets the need. Force on the other hand, is exhausted. Force goes from here to there. It extends its own energy.

You have to constantly stoke force with more and more energy. Money, bodies of soldiers, bodies of believers, their gold, their lives, their sweat—you have to pull it out. The Roman empire, which was the greatest empire the world had ever seen, petered out after a thousand years. So force is limited; power, on the other hand, is unlimited.

TRUTH AND SUBJECTIVITY

When you define what is truth, it's impossible to define truth without defining the context. And that is the reason all the greatest philosophers that have ever lived have never solved the problems of epistemology, because they never got that subtlety. You move from the objective to the subjective. The objective will take you up to 499 (on the Map of Consciousness), and from there you move into the subjective. The presence of God is not something one can experience through thought, but experientially, it is subjective.

What kinesiology, or consciousness calibration, shows us is that consciousness itself recognizes the presence of truth. At first, I thought it was truth versus falsehood. I thought consciousness knows the truth from the false.

Actually, consciousness itself recognizes the presence of truth. It only knows the truth and the not true. It knows what's true and fails to recognize what is not true. You see how that gets us out of polarity—you see how there's a subtlety to this? It gets you out of the spiritual guilt of the polarity of the opposites, where you like this and hate that, and you feel guilty because you're supposed to be spiritual and not hate anything.

See, there's chocolate and vanilla. You can like chocolate without hating vanilla. You don't have to hate vanilla, you can just choose chocolate. You can be conservative and not hate the liberals because they're all vanilla. They can be vanilla liberals. And they don't have to hate conservatives because they're chocolate. They can just like vanilla, and say to themselves, *I don't know how you digest that chocolate, but that's your problem, you know?* One chocolate guy says, "Vanilla is for wimps. If you like vanilla, you like vanilla. But us guys, we like chocolate." You can champion your cause. You can tell others that we're the greatest, and tattoo yourself, and make parades, and all that. But you don't have to get into hate.

CALIBRATING THE CONSCIOUSNESS LEVEL OF MANKIND

The purpose of our discussion, of course, is to potentiate the evolution of consciousness. And the only purpose of the books I've written or the lectures I've given is to support the progression of that consciousness within the individual who has elected to pursue a higher level of consciousness.

Most people think they're in the ordinary world of causality. They think that what they are is the product of their past. The reality is that it's the *potentiality* of what you have chosen to become that is pulling you into the present. So if you're reading this book, it's not because what you've been in the past is pushing you up to this point. On the contrary, it's because you elected to be that which is beyond this point that is pulling you through this point. It's because you have *chosen* already by spiritual intention.

People often ask, "What's karma about?" Well, karma is just the automatic energy consequent of spiritual intention and spiritual decision. Every decision you make then affects your calibrated level of consciousness, which is another way of saying your *karma*. It starts first as curiosity, and next thing you know, you find yourself automatically drawn into spiritual growth and spiritual concepts and the desire to understand them and to benefit from them. You begin to realize that as you grow, you're benefiting the world; that what you're doing is affecting everyone. The whole world benefits from you. We can prove that also with quantum mechanics, the Heisenberg principle, and the collapse of the wave function that then begins to affect the whole field of consciousness. Every individual who commits to spiritual work is benefiting all of humanity. This is an automatic consequence of his choices and decisions, because he's collapsing the potential into the actual, which is impacting the collective consciousness of all mankind.

We found it quite interesting when we were calibrating levels of consciousness. We asked: What is the level of consciousness of mankind? Well, that led to a rather major discovery. We found that the consciousness of mankind throughout the ages has been constantly, slowly, very slowly, progressing. At the time of the birth of Buddha, the consciousness level of mankind was 90. At the time of the birth of Jesus Christ, the consciousness level of mankind was 100. Then down through the ages this slowly evolved, and through the 1200s, 1400s, and 1700s, it stayed at 190. It stayed at 190 century after century—didn't move. Then suddenly in the late 1980s, at about the time of the Harmonic Convergence—not caused by it, but at the time of it—and at the time of the collapse of Monolithic Communism and many other things, the consciousness level jumped from 190 to 207. Now, 200 is the level of truth; 200 is the level of integrity. It is probably the most significant event in the history of mankind. Unnoticed, the shift of consciousness went from 190 to 207. That completely changes the field in which all of us now live.

So, how does it change mankind? Well, at 190, the destruction of all mankind was inevitable. The great mega bomb that was going to destroy all life was a considerable likelihood. At 207 now, there's a whole new paradigm of reality. In the world in which I grew up, in the 1930s and on through that century, the goal of life was success. You were supposed to make money, be successful, go to college, get a name for yourself, and so on.

Now at 207, people are not interested in your success. I mean, you can buy some stock and be a millionaire tomorrow, and so what? No, now what we're looking at is integrity. All the great corporations whose heads have rolled have been criticized for lack of integrity. We see politicians being called to task for integrity. Success and money and having a big car and all the stuff that used to make people happy in the '50s no longer suffices. Now people are asking, *What is the integrity of this company? What is the integrity of this politician?* We're looking at how truthful they are. How can they back up their statements? Integrity is the new signal of social value. We want to invest in people and politicians and teachers who have a proven integrity.

How can you prove it? Well, one way you can prove it is, frankly, by calibrating its level. That which is integrous then has a value. Integrity has power. Lack of integrity can have force, monetary force, for a moment, but it collapses, which is why you can't base your life on success. Therefore, the new paradigm of value is integrity, and it's by integrity now that everyone is going to be measured. *How integrous of a teacher are you? How integrous is this spiritual mentor or organization?* And when you calibrate all these things, you see where integrity is sold out.

We've calibrated many, many things, so you can see where any compromise in integrity shows up on the dotted line. Because you can now measure it, and calibrate truth from falsehood, I think we will have a new yardstick by which to measure man's growth, and he will grow faster than before. We saw for centuries it stayed at 190, no movement; though from a historical viewpoint, people say great events happened. (Great events from a perceptual viewpoint, not from a spiritual viewpoint.)

Man is now in a new dimension, and 207 is critical because it only takes one feather to tip the balance from negative to positive. Every spiritual decision we make can tip the scale to the positive side, and that totally changes the destiny of our life. If you're out at sea, a change of one degree in the compass may not seem like much, but after a couple of days of sailing, you'll end up on a different continent. So one degree makes quite a bit of difference. Freedom of choice, then—spiritual choice—is what we're confronted with instant by instant. Instant by instant, we're constantly saying yes or no to choices. And those choices then determine our spiritual level and our calibrated level of consciousness and our karmic destiny.

THE DUALITY OF THE EGO

This discovery led to my eventually becoming a spiritual teacher. I wanted to share my own subjective state and things that have never really been said before. What I teach, I call *devotional non-duality*. Devotional because one is in love with the truth. One is in love with the pathway to God through truth. And non-duality, meaning that to reach a state of enlightenment, one has to transcend the ego. The ego is dualistic in nature. Human thinking is dualistic in nature. There's an either or, this or that. The spiritual student is usually confronted. It starts first with confronting the ego and what has traditionally been called sin (and given all kinds of bad names).

The first thing I wanted my students to understand is the nature of the ego and to become friendly with it, and understand where it comes from. You have to get away from demonizing it. You can't see it as an enemy. The ego is nothing but the animal nature. When you look at the animal kingdom, all you see is what's called the human ego. When we see it in an animal, we just say, "It's nature." But when we see it in a human, we say, "Oh, isn't that awful?" No, it's not awful.

With evolution, we see the emergence of the mammalian brain from the reptilian brain, and for the first time, we see the emergence of love. Love didn't emerge on this planet for millions of years, not until the mammalian brain. When we see a mother bird caring for her eggs and baby birds, it's really the mammalian brain that we begin to see. So, we don't see love until we see really the emergence of the maternal instinct. Love doesn't appear until we see the mother's concern for the child, the infant, the fledgling. We don't see it arising primarily early in the evolution of the animal world.

Love begins to emerge as the expression of the maternal; then you begin to see love blossom over the ages. Romantic love, which we take for granted in today's world, is a rather recent occurrence. For many centuries, people didn't get married for romantic love; it was a transfer of power. They got married because the family arranged it. The kings and queens of England, for all their power, weren't free to choose love. They figured marriage is one thing, love is another. So romantic love, as we see it, is a rather recent and modern thing.

When people go into spiritual work, they are always concerned about overcoming the ego. So first we say, recontextualize it as the residual of the animal within us. The old animal brain is still present in the back of the human brain, and the prefrontal cortex is a rather recent emergence. If you calibrate the level of consciousness of hominids, as they evolved over time, you see Cro-Magnon, you see Neanderthal. A Neanderthal calibrates around 75 (on the Map), a really animalistic level. Although it's able to speak and talk, it's still pretty much an animal. It's only with the emergence of the forebrain and the prefrontal cortex that you begin to see ethics, morality, spiritual awareness, and so on. What humans are trying to do, then, is transcend domination by their animal instincts. It helps if you take the ego out of the viewpoint of *sin* and begin to see it as *animal*. What is an animal like? Well, you can see the human ego on display at any zoo. Go to the monkey island in the zoo and you see territoriality, you see gangs; they hang together in groups and then fight over turf.

There are always turf wars going on around the world. Then you see the exploitation or the subjugation of the weak. You see deception and lying and camouflage, and so all you see in today's headlines is the monkey island with a human expression.

Spiritual work is really about overcoming selfishness, self-centeredness, and egocentricity in all of its various disguises. What are the various disguises? Well, the compulsion to have, to own, to be successful, to win, and all the things that we know as egocentricity. How does one then begin to transcend that? People say, "Well, I'm interested in evolving spiritually. What can I do from a practical viewpoint?" Because all what I've just described can sound quite advanced and quite theoretical and quite imposing to somebody who's not familiar with the work.

Actually, this work becomes rather easy; the more you practice, the more you arrive at the feeling of *I knew this all along.* Of course, you did know it all along, but you want to know how to transform this feeling in everyday life. So people say, "How can I grow spiritually? Do I have to go somewhere? Do I have to get a guru? Do I have to join a meditation group? Do I have to recite mantras or what?"

No, you don't have to do that at all.

It's so simple that it's overlooked all the time. It's a decision to be loving and kind toward all life, including your own, at all times, no matter what. To be forgiving, to be gentle, to be that which is supportive of life. So that becomes not what you *do*, but what you *are*. You become that which supports life, supports all endeavors. It encourages those who need encouragement, and it becomes the energy of life itself. It becomes almost like the manifestation of the Divine Mother, as well as the Divine Father, so it's the merging of the two: that which is nurturing and that which is demanding of excellence.

It's so simple that it's overlooked all the time. It's a decision to be loving and kind toward all of life, including your own, at all times, no matter what. To be forgiving, to be gentle, to be that which is supportive of life.

STARTING ON THE PATHWAY OF NON-DUALITY

The pathway of non-duality, then, is the devotion to spiritual principles, and as you become devoted to spiritual principles, you're brought up face-to-face with the mind's propensity for either/or: good or evil, liberal or conservative. You're confronted constantly with the so-called polarities, and to reach a very advanced state of consciousness, it is then necessary to transcend the so-called polarities of either/or-ness.

The ego would have you think that it's responsible for your survival. Ego says, "If I wasn't so clever . . . if I didn't remind you to take your vitamins and all, you'd be deader than a mackerel." The downside of duality, then, is it creates the illusion that there's a separate *I* that is the cause of everything—that there's a personal *I*, separate from the infinite oneness of totality. The core of the ego is this self-centered point, which one assumes to be the cause of everything. As long as you believe in causality, you are stuck in a duality of "a this causing a that." The pathway to enlightenment through non-duality dissolves the opposites.

The ego is so impressed by popularity, wanting to be right, vanity, and pridefulness. Give up the vanity of wanting to be right. Spirituality is really a way of being in the world. People think of spirituality in terms of the ego's function, of *doingness*. It's not a *doingness*, however, it's a way of *beingness* in the world. It's a way of being with the world in which one is in a constant state of appreciation and service. Why? Because you become discerning of the beauty of existence, to become benign, to be cordial, to be loving toward all things. If I had not felt loving toward that rattlesnake, which I will talk about in Chapter 5, I would never have lived long enough to tell you the tale. The respect for all that exists. Truly spiritual people are willing to see the intrinsic beauty of all of existence. To be benign and to be unconditionally loving toward all things, at all times.

If you want to become spiritually evolved, it's very simple. Let's say the ideal is, *I wish to see the world the way it is.* And the only way to see it, the way it is, is to decide to be loving toward all, no matter what—to be respectful and loving toward all that exists. To be committed to life in all its expressions, to discern the beauty and perfection of all that exists, is a way of being in the world. So, as I said, it's not a *doingness*, it's a *beingness*. To make rapid spiritual advancement, you make a decision to *be* that which fulfills the potential of life and to witness its beauty and perfection and all of its expressions.

The ego sees everything in terms of cause; it sees everything as going from imperfection to perfection, from incomplete to complete. With spiritual vision, you begin to see everything is going from perfection to perfection. Everything is moving from perfection, and everything is already complete at the moment. Everything is completely what it is, as the consequence of the evolution of creation up to this point. And you see that everything is moving, not from incomplete, but from complete to complete, from perfection to perfection. This is a perfect cut on the back of my hand. It's a perfect expression of what happens as a perfect scab forms, and then it'll get to be a perfect healing, and it'll leave a perfect scar. Everything is being perfectly what it's destined to be, and fulfilling its potential. So instead of causality, what you begin to see is emergence. The world is not a world of cause at all.

Everything is moving from perfection, and everything is already complete at the moment. Everything is completely what it is, as the consequence of the evolution of creation up to this point.

We live in a world of *emergence*. Everything, every instant has a certain potentiality. So you begin to see that things are not happening due to causality, not due to a personal self. You see the emergence of potentiality into actuality. The fulfillment as the rose blooms and becomes a full rose—nothing is causing it, nothing is forcing it, and nothing is even deciding it. The potentiality to open fully, open its petals, already resides within the rose every instant. It's not an imperfect rose half opened; it's a rose that's perfectly half opened. So there you transform your experience of life and the world and reality, by seeing that everything is perfect every instant. People ask me, "How can you improve this world?" I tell them not to bother. This world is perfect the way it is. There's no point in trying to improve the world, because the world you see, it doesn't even exist. If the purpose of the world is karmic benefit and evolution of consciousness, then this world is perfect as it is. This is a very high, spiritual understanding.

Chapter 2

CALIBRATION

Now that you have the ideas, inspiration, and encouragement to begin walking the path of enlightenment, how do you determine the steps to take in order to stay on this path? And how can you be sure that you're progressing along the path, and not simply walking in circles?

Dr. Hawkins used a well-known method and developed a breakthrough spiritual tool to help answer these questions. The method he used was that of kinesiology, in order to calibrate spiritual truth from falsehood, so one could be sure that he or she was following the precepts of a person of integrity, for example, rather than a wolf in sheep's clothing.

Using this method of calibration, Dr. Hawkins developed his Map of Consciousness, which outlines calibrated levels of consciousness from 0 to 1,000, essentially providing a map in which to progress up the enlightenment path.

In this chapter, Dr. Hawkins explains the calibration method and the Map of Consciousness, so you can reach the very highest levels of enlightenment.

It's a biological fact that truth makes your body go strong, and falsehood makes it go weak. You don't have to label it anything; it's just a matter of fact. If I hold that which is negative in mind, and somebody tests the strength of my arm muscles, they will go weak. Moreover, if I hold something uplifting, true, and of a high calibration in mind, the arm goes strong.

Now, *I* don't have anything to do with that. That's a physiologic response. In the lectures, I give the reason for this. The likely reasons are evolutionary—that animal life does not have within it a source of energy. Plant life has chlorophyll. It just sits in the sun and absorbs energy. It doesn't have to acquire or get. Animal life is protoplasmic. It does not have within it any source of energy. It has to acquire it. In order to survive, animal life—protoplasmic life, of which humans are, of course, an example—has to be able to find out what is nutritious and helpful and life-sustaining.

So the first thing the amoeba has to learn is what will increase its strength and survival, and what will kill it. It therefore has to learn, at a very low level of consciousness, what is pro-life and what is anti-life. What is pro-life makes you strong, vigorous. You multiply and are successful. And if you don't have the capacity, you die. You only have to make one mistake, confusing what's nutritious and what's poisonous. You don't get a second chance to relearn, because those who didn't learn are dead.

Consequently, the only reason humans are here is because we learned that. If we hadn't learned that, we would've been dead a long time ago. So, protoplasmic entities that fail to learn how to differentiate truth from falsehood, poisonous from nutritious, don't survive. The fact that any kind of organism is still living means it has within it, innately, some capacity to discern that which is pro-life from that which is anti-life. If it didn't, it would be dead.

The people in Europe who could not differentiate a dictator who was malevolent from a great leader who was beneficial lost their lives. To not know the difference between that which calibrates over 200 and that which calibrates extremely below 200, cost 10 million lives. In my lifetime, in Europe, 10 million people died. If you hold Hitler in mind, and try to hold your arm straight parallel to the ground, you'll find you're weak. You can hardly hold up a small book. If you hold Jesus Christ in mind, your arm is powerfully strong. If you hold Churchill in mind, your arm goes strong. And if you hold Stalin in mind, your arm goes weak.

Now, this is true even if you don't know anything about the person. Let's say I take a picture of this person, and I hold it in mind. The way I do the test is I ask the person whose arm I'm using. I don't want to influence their response in any way, so I'll say, "What I'm holding in mind calibrates as true." Then, I press down. If it's true, their arm goes strong. If it's false, it goes weak.

Or I could say, "It calibrates over 200. Yes? Yes? No. Calibrates over 300. Yes, no. Okay." So, what is true, then, is life-sustaining, and what is life-sustaining, through the acupuncture energy system, in the acupuncture meridians, makes your body go strong instantly. Once you learn how to approach it, you know how to handle it, like anything else. Just because you understand physiology doesn't mean you can go without oxygen at 10,000 feet. You can't. Once you understand the basic principles, muscle testing is extremely easy.

THE IMPORTANCE OF INTEGRITY IN CALIBRATION

Now, about 10 percent of the population cannot use this method, for reasons we don't know yet—maybe karmic reasons. People under consciousness level 200 cannot use it with any degree of accuracy. They have to be integrous, and the intention of the question has to be integrous. If you're going to use the technique to find the best way to rob the bank, you're not going to get reliable answers!

Let's say you want to donate money to a fund, and you ask, "This fund is integrous, yes, no?" And then if you get a yes, you say, "It's over 200, 300, 400. How integrous is this organization?" And then once you know all that, you see there are some organizations that sound like the greatest philanthropies in the world, but they must spend billions of dollars on advertising. And when you calibrate them, it makes your arm go weak. If the fund was truly integrous, it would make your arm go strong, would it not?

Each person is different. I look at it pragmatically, and I use muscle testing to solve things that are not readily apparent, or to confirm something that I presume is apparent, but I want to make sure that I'm not misperceiving it. So, you use it sporadically. Sometimes you use it intensely. When I'm doing research, I use it rather intensely. If I'm diagnosing today's world, I want to calibrate every politician out there, every big-time spokesman, everybody who gets on there with a big spiel, and people's stories and excuses.

I say, "What's the energy of this candidate? This candidate tells this story. Is that so? All right, this candidate hung out with so and so. What does *that* person calibrate at?" I get a whole picture of multiple aspects, because pretty soon what happens is a whole picture begins to fill in. Your whole movie set fills in. First you get the walls, then you get the carpet, then your pictures on the walls and the various actors. And the picture begins to fit in, and then the storyline becomes quite obvious—why this person said this at this time. And you constantly verify.

Now, people also change. So, you may see a change in a prominent person. And you can ask, "Is this person still at the same level? Or has this one been bought out?" You have to be prepared to find out things you're not going to like.

Of course, don't forget: the more often you do this, the more things you calibrate, the more experience you have, the greater your degree of accuracy. After you've done it 10,000 times, you could look at almost anything and know what it's going to calibrate at within a couple degrees.

It's a great learning tool. You learn a lot about your own consciousness. You learn a lot about your own motivations. You're not going to get an accurate answer, unless you can remove your own personal prejudice of wanting this answer or that answer. Somebody that you think is a scurrilous, horrible person, you find out that they calibrate over 200. Somebody else that you think is going to be the savior of the world, you find out they're under 200, that they're actually full of hot wind. They're a very adept politician, but a good politician is different than a statesman.

Generally speaking, Americans don't appreciate the difference. To them, a politician and a statesman are one and the same. They're quite different, and they calibrate quite differently. The politician is interested in *me, me, me,* and is very glib. They get what they want for their own personal gain. A statesman is what he is for the sake of the world and the sake of the country. An example is Winston Churchill: Britain would've been beaten senseless if it wasn't for Winston. He calibrated 500.

GETTING STARTED

You can do muscle testing by yourself. On your left hand, touch your middle finger and your thumb so that they make an O. Now, with your right hand, take your forefinger and hook it inside the O. Try to pull the middle finger and thumb apart. Now, if something is true, you'll find it takes a lot of effort to try and break that O. If what you're holding in mind is negative, you'll find it's weak.

Muscle testing can also be conducted with multiple people. Here's how: hold your right arm or your left arm out parallel with the ground. Now, have somebody else press down on your wrist with two fingers—maybe four, five ounces of pressure. We're not trying to break the arm down. As always, the accuracy of this method depends on the consciousness level of the participants. If you're both over 200, then the likelihood is you'll get an accurate result. Remember: both participants have to be integrous to begin with.

What does *integrous* really mean, anyway? It means that you're more interested in the truth than trying to prove some preconsidered notion. So, if I hold something that has a negative energy against the solar plexus of a person with their arm stretched out to the side and press down on their wrist, their arm will fall down. Their arm will drop. They're very weak. If I think about certain kinds of music such as types of heavy metal or rap, or pesticides, or anything that's negative—there's a whole lot of things—within the aura of the person being tested, and I press down, their arm will go weak. Conversely, if I hold something or someone in mind that is positive, their arm will go strong.

Now, the difference is quite marked. The person who's very strong will be very strong, and with two fingers, you're not going to push them down. And with something that makes them go weak, a child could push them down with two fingers. When they go weak, they go weak. So, for instance, if I take a volume by Plato or Socrates and hold it against the solar plexus, the person goes strong. If I take *The Communist Manifesto* and hold it against their stomach, their arm goes weak. Karl Marx calibrates at 130.

You might ask, "How do you know Marx's calibration level?" Well, Marx calibrates over 110, 120, 130. When I get to 130, that's the end of the yes and no. Does he calibrate over 130? The answer is no.

I can do the same thing with President Reagan. I can do it with Abraham Lincoln. I can do it with the great pyramids in Egypt. I can do it with anything on the planet. Truth makes you go strong; falsehood makes you weak.

So, this has a biologic basis. The capacity to discern essence from appearance is essential for life. If a bacterium doesn't know the difference between that which is poisonous and that which is nutritious, it will soon die . . . and there won't be any bacteria left. Survival depends, from a protoplasmic point of view, on the capacity to discern that which is pro-life from that which is anti-life. And falsehood is anti-life, and truth is pro-life.

It's like riding a bicycle. It takes some experience. Some people are quite adept at it. First of all, they take my word for what I say as absolute truth, and don't put up a lot of doubt blocks and quizzicalness. If I say it works, it works. If it didn't work, why would I say it works? You have to have a certain trust in the authenticity of people.

I share the muscle testing method with people because it's extremely helpful. There are societies in which it is very common. When I was in the East, it was *very* common. You'd see a person shopping, holding a tomato in his hand, pressing down on it, and if it went weak it was not a good tomato. Some people incorporate it into their culture. The fact that truth makes you strong and falsehood makes you weak seems to be such basic common sense, you wouldn't think that intellectual people would argue with it.

Let's say I'm the person who's doing the testing, and my partner is resisting, and I'm pressing down with two fingers. I don't want to influence that person's thinking or tip them off to what I'm thinking. With integrous people, you could say it out loud and it's not going to affect them. But most people are not that integrous. So what I'll say is, "What I'm holding in mind calibrates over 100, 150, 200, 250, 300," until I get a yes from the participant. That way, I'm not influencing the answer, because the person whose arm I'm pressing down on doesn't know what I'm holding in my mind. I don't want to contaminate the answer.

I'm not going to waste my time getting a false answer, either. People think, *Oh, you're out to get a false answer.* Why would I waste my time getting a false answer, chasing my own tail for amusement? I don't think it's very entertaining. I want to make it count. So I say, "Now, what I'm holding in mind . . . calibrates over so and so," such as political candidates or programs. I don't influence the response, because I myself want to know the answer. If both participants want to know what is the truth for truth's sake, then you're going to have a successful team.

Like anything, it takes a little practice. Some things will blow you out, like the negative heavy metal music we tested. I suggest turning off music, television, and other distractions. There's all kinds of negative energies coming through, so you're going to get false negatives. That's because of the background energy of the sounds, so you've got to turn those off.

To help resolve doubt, and all the controversies and gossip and all, often I will get up and say, "This guy calibrates over so and so. I wonder where he's coming from. He sounds like about 160 to me." Well, he was coming from 160. In other words, I want to confirm my own impression. So, there's perception and then there's *essence.*

So what I do is I use calibration to confirm the essence of a thing—that I'm not just falling for perception. Because a smooth talker can sound pretty persuasive when you first encounter them.

You say, "Boy, that sounds like a swell guy." And then you do the arm test, and he comes out 180. You say, "Oh. What's the answer? Now I've got a problem." It's when perception does not match essence that I use it to calibrate unknown factors, and I want a quick idea of how integrous this thing is.

If you don't have any idea what a thing is altogether, say, "This is above 200 or this is below 200." Or "This is above 200," to give you some idea of the range of it. You get pretty perspicacious after you've done a few thousand of these. I can usually guess the number within a couple of points. You're training your intuition. It's an area of life we don't usually train, because we have no way to check its veracity, usually.

But by constantly calibrating things, as I say, you become pretty skilled at it. I'd say at least nine out of ten times, you're at least within the ballpark of what the reality is. The average person is not. The average person is pretty easy to fool. They like to pride themselves on the fact they can't be deceived, but the statistics show that the contrary is true.

CALIBRATION, ATHEISTS, AND NARCISSISM

Well-known professors pooh-poohed this method, and it doesn't work for atheists. If you negate the truth, the reality of the truth of God, which is one of the aspects of divinity, then you become disallowed and disenfranchised from using the methodology. Therefore, an atheist cannot use it. I don't want them to waste time trying it. That takes you out of the ring right to begin with.

The people who argue with it are often atheists. You'll find that atheists hate this method, because they hate absolutism. They want everything to be relativism. The idea that there is an absolute to whom one is answerable is an antonym. God is confrontational to the narcissism of the ego. The ego's narcissism is unbridled. It will disavow God. It's *greater* than God.

Here's Joe Blow down from nowhere, who's in his sophomore year in college, and he already "knows" that there is no divinity. He calibrates at 192, and divinity calibrates at infinity. So here's this one guy at 192, refuting the reality of that which calibrates at *infinity*. There are no limits to the expansiveness of the human ego.

The atheist is tied into a belief system, but the primary motive behind it is narcissism. The primary motive behind it is naivete. They're unaware that the intellect, which calibrates in the 400s, is not in the paradigm to even consider spiritual realities, which are 500 and up. You can't prove or disprove canoeing on the basketball court. And I tell people who don't believe in my work, "Don't believe in it!" I have no interest in whether they believe it or not. Who cares if they believe it or not? I can tell you which way I found is east, and if you want to go your own way, you can go your own way. But I know which way is east—that's all.

Some people don't understand that I am obligated to speak the truth. I'm not saying this for the listener. I'm saying it because I'm responsible, and I am answerable to God. It's because I'm answerable to God that I give you the truth as I understand it. It's because I'm *accountable* to divinity. A person who doesn't believe in divinity is accountable to no one except the narcissistic core of his own ego. People who are more spiritually evolved realize that at the moment of death's door, they're about to become answerable, in capital letters. They're going to either notice something with devils with horns or tails, or they're going to hear angels singing.

THE CALIBRATED MAP OF CONSCIOUSNESS

Through muscle testing, then, I discovered a phenomenon, and that phenomenon then allowed for calibrating the levels of consciousness. The phenomenon is innate to life. Out of this arose a calibrated Map of Consciousness, a logarithmic scale, one to 1,000, which includes all possibility within this domain, with 1,000 being the level of the great avatars: Jesus Christ, Buddha, Krishna, Zoroaster. It's as high as you can go in this domain. Why? Because human protoplasm can't handle energies beyond that. In fact, from about 800 and up, it's very difficult for the nervous system to handle that kind of energy. It gets very uncomfortable in the 800s—often quite painful and agonizing at times.

If your consciousness goes beyond 1,000, you belong in a different realm, and you leave here. You can hear your protoplasm sizzling in the sun, and it's time to let go of the protoplasmic. So, because of the limitations of the human nervous system and protoplasm, the Map of Consciousness only goes up to 1,000.

Archangels calibrate at such high frequencies. The one who once noticed me calibrated at 50,000, and a passing notice changed my life completely. It was like a devastating shot of lightning. So, just pray that no archangel really thinks about you too much. Higher isn't always better.

Descartes said man doesn't know whether reality is what he perceives is reality. There's res interna and then there's res externa. The world the way it is or nature itself. And of course, Socrates, who's my favorite old teacher, said the same thing. All men are innocent by virtue of the fact that they're unable to discern appearance from essence, truth from falsehood, and that they pursue illusion. They always pursue what they perceive to be the good.

That helps us put in place, then, forgiveness, or Christ's statement, that the only human error is one of ignorance. People make errors, and the innocence of the child still resides within all of us. That's why we are dupable and programmable; like the child, the mind tends to believe everything that it hears.

Of course, what we learn through this technique is devastating. What actually goes on in the world, as compared to its appearance, is quite remarkable. Although the world doesn't know what's going on, we do within a matter of seconds. The whole world studies the thing, and doesn't even know what it's about!

Remember: only people who themselves calibrate over 200 can use the technique, and only if their intention is integrous. You can't use the technique to try and prove a point—to try and get the world to agree with you. You have to be dedicated to truth for its own sake. And then when you find out the truth, you can worry about what to do about it later. But the first thing is, you don't know what the problem is until you ask what the truth of the matter is. Our dedication is to truth, and the basis is that truth is the straight way to God. And nonlinear duality means to let go of the linear appearance of things, and to align with the essence, which is the fastest way to enlightenment.

The view of God, then, depends on your level of consciousness—whether you see God as punitive or frightening, or whether you're an atheist and don't believe in God at all. Your view of yourself depends on your level of consciousness. It doesn't depend on sociologic conditions, poverty, or wealth, or any of these things. Your view of yourself is a consequence of your own level of consciousness.

We gave these levels useful names. The spiritualization of these levels go all the way from enlightenment, down to the high levels—600 is a phenomenal level. In the human domain, very few people get to 500. Fewer yet get to unconditional love, at 540. In the world's population, 0.4 percent ever reaches unconditional love. People ask, "How can I reach unconditional love?" I say, "Well, become an alcoholic and join AA. It's at 540." Or you can study *A Course in Miracles*.

These ways all depend on simplicity and the willingness to be forgiving—the willingness to live one day at a time. You put them into your life and daily application, to make them part of your life. That means you have to give up the pleasure of condemning people.

Reason is at the 400s. Love is 500. There's unconditional love, and *beyond* unconditional love. We start out with shame, disaster, guilt, apathy, fear, and anger. This level of 200 is very critical. At level 200, we have the willingness to be honest. Self-honesty is the only requirement of any of these spiritual programs. Self-honesty automatically puts you above level 200.

From here up, you're interested in the truth for its own sake. And what happens here is extremely important, because the brain chemistry shifts. You shift from left brain, animal, instinctual dominance of the ego. The Kundalini energy arises, and you now shift to right brain, which sees things in a benign way, processes information differently, and also releases neurotransmitters and neurohormones that alter the way your brain physiology works.

People hoping that everybody in the world's going to get together and sing songs and join hands, and that we're all going to be happy, are forgetting that the people below 200 have a different brain physiology, and, frankly, to them you sound like an idiot. So all the do-gooder peaceniks who want to envision a new, peaceful world are forgetting that 85 percent of the world calibrates below 200. In America, approximately 50 percent. And these people have a different brain physiology. This means that what you're saying to them is nonsensical, meaningless, and probably absurd, and for which, in their minds, you actually deserve to be killed.

That makes it a little difficult—how are you going to turn this into one peaceful world? People are always asking, "What can I do to help the world?" Well, being quiet and minding your own business are a good start! Why? Because what actually helps the world is your personal spiritual evolution. *That's* what helps the world. Your kindness to others begins to lift the overall level of consciousness of mankind, which unfortunately was up high and now it's come down again.

As we know, the consciousness level of mankind was at 190 for many, many thousands of years. At the time of Jesus Christ, it was at about 100. It slowly came up to 190, and it stayed at 190 over the centuries, through the 1800s and early 1900s. And then in the late '80s, at the time of the Harmonic Concordance or Convergence, it suddenly jumped to 205. And it stayed at 205. The next time there was a Harmonic Concordance or Convergence, we were giving a lecture in San Francisco. And at the exact time of this event, consciousness level of mankind went from 205 to 207. This was documented and recorded: it went to 207.

Since that time, it stayed steady, and then it slowly started to decrease again. So it was at 207, then it came down 206, 205, and now it's come down to 204, which is a little close to the line, because 200 is really the critical line, due to two things: the effect of the philosophy of relativism, and all of its invasion of integrity and truth, together with the people dedicated to violence. So between violence on one side, and apologists for the violent people on the other side, the world has come down.

But that's not really our concern. We'll let God worry about that. The world is perfect as it is. It offers the maximum karmic potential of choice. The spirit cannot evolve unless it has choice. If you're forced to always be a certain way, there's no karmic merit.

Because you take the responsibility for the evolution of your own consciousness, every second you are making choices. The human spirit is sort of like a karmic track. I always picture that it's like a little, tiny iron filing, and the infinite field of consciousness is like an infinitely powerful electromagnetic field, so that by virtue of that which you have become, you position yourself within the field.

There's no judgmental God who says you're being bad and you're being good. No one says if you're good, we'll reward you and move you over here, and if you're bad, we'll put you down here. You have your own choice; nobody steers your canoe but you. You, by your own choices and by your own agreement, more or less, change the charges on yourself. Let's look at this in terms of positive and negative. I'll say, "You're an SOB, and I hate you," and then you go a little more negative. And then you say, "But I forgive you," and then you go a little more positive.

You probably didn't know what you were doing, like Socrates said. On the other hand, you ought to know by now, and move on a little bit. So, you see, you're like a little thing like this, fluctuating in the electromagnetic spectrum. And the spirit is what survives, and when it leaves the body, it goes to that which it is.

So, I agree with Freud that the negative depictions of God are projections from the human unconscious. However, Freud then went on and made a mistake. He went further than that. He said, "Therefore, a true God doesn't exist." No. Just because a false God doesn't exist, doesn't mean a true one doesn't. So, that's why Freud calibrated 499.

The 400s are extremely powerful and important. Love is 500; joy is 540. And as you reach the higher levels, you find unconditional love, which, I think, is the best goal to aim for in human life. Unconditional love is reachable within the human domain. The states of enlightenment are very difficult to reach in today's world, but unconditional love means that you leave and you move into heavenly and celestial realms.

If you want to save the world, I would suggest the first thing you do is let go and surrender the world to God, which is the same thing other great teachers have said. The world that you see doesn't even exist. It's all a projection of your own perception. You can let go of wanting to change it, because all you're changing is your own projections that you've projected out there. You're not changing anything in the world at all.

Unless a man has a choice between good and evil, how's he going to transcend? If you don't have any enemies, who do you have left to forgive? You know what I mean? *I'm a failure. I haven't got anybody I'd love to forgive. Now, what are we going to do in the Course in Miracles?*

Spiritual work is primarily yin. It's yang by its intention, but it's yin by its operation. For example, I ask God what is the answer to a thing, and then I step back and allow the space for revelation. So, progress is achieved often without even thinking—you just have a feeling of knowing or an intuition. And then if you know muscle testing, you can just check it out for affirmation. It has been very, very useful.

The enlightened and divined states, the supreme God and all these things, calibrate at 1,000 or above. As we know, the majority of the world's population calibrates below 200. Why doesn't the world go to pieces and just destroy itself? It gets close to that periodically. Mankind has been at war 93 percent of recorded time. The other 7 percent, we were too sick or too poor, probably. The plague was on. Couldn't get our act together to get out there and kill each other.

Why doesn't the world just self-destruct? It's because it's a logarithmic scale. So logarithmically, the advance of a few points is enormously powerful. In fact, in the United States, even just a couple of people calibrate so high and logarithmically, the power is so great that it totally counterbalances the negativity of mankind, which would self-destruct. So, those who are 200 and up—readers like you—are keeping the world from going down the tubes.

The relative power, because it's logarithmic, is so enormous that it counterbalances the negativity.

LOWER LEVELS OF CONSCIOUSNESS

Now, I just want to show the source of the evil of the ego. Because you see, consciousness began at a very primitive level, the consciousness level. Over many billions of years, the consciousness level slowly rose. The consciousness level of life itself, the total consciousness of life on the planet, has evolved over billions of years, very, very slowly.

Sometimes the consciousness level of the animals has kept it up. Even though man has been lower than 200 many times, there are many animals on the planet that are over 200. Somebody says, "Well, the consciousness level of man is at about 204. How come you've got life at 212?" It's because we got kitties and doggies. A dog's wagging a tail is at 500.

I didn't want to say anything that might hurt people's feelings. But cats and dogs do better than people. Chimpanzees and gorillas, too. You're safer with Koko the gorilla than you are with most of the people on the subway. Koko won't steal your purse and run. Monkeys, dogs, cats. Of course, the more cats you have, the higher your level of consciousness. I'm a cat supporter. Our level of consciousness at home, without the cats, would probably collapse.

Let's not forget horses, elephants, and cows. These are all primarily herbivores. When you see how life starts out, at the lowest level, and that we come up through fish, octopus, the Komodo dragon, and other predatory mammals, you see that life is voracious. Below consciousness level 200, it only can survive by eating others. And then, as the consciousness level goes higher, you get to the herbivores.

At consciousness level 200, we have wolves and foxes. Then, all of a sudden, at the level 200, we shift to zebras, giraffes, deer, bison, domestic pigs, elk, cows, and sheep. Do you see the shift? You eat grass and you're not harming anybody; whereas the dinosaur has to kill. He has to kill in order to eat. His nature is to kill.

The dinosaur is not being bad or evil, that's just his nature. He's reflecting the level of consciousness. So the people on the planet who seem to be focused on killing do so because their level of consciousness is attuned to be less than 200. Therefore, the left brain, the instinctual left brain physiology, takes over, in which killing becomes exciting, fun, and rewarding.

We talked about the 400s being, you might say, when humans reach their greatest intellectual excellence, probably around 350 BC. In ancient Greece, philosophically, there really hasn't been any improvement since that time. And here we calibrate the great books of the Western world, and we find it's very interesting. Overall, collectively it calibrates around 460. So intellectual excellence, intellectual truth, and reason are in the 400s. In the old days, a liberal education meant to study all of these writers. And there is still a foundation for the study of the Great Books. They advise you to take 10 years. So you spend 10 years studying, and you will then share a common understanding with all the greatest minds that've ever lived—at least within the intellectual and philosophic realms.

So, the difficulty of something of a very low calibration is that this then starts off a trend that becomes self-propagating, in the form of memes. An infection like this can then spread throughout the world. People ask me, "How can I become spiritual?" Well, I say, "First, just become a decent human being. Try that. Be considerate, decent. Be responsible. If you say you're going to close the door when you leave, please do so." People have to be able to count on you. You have to be honest and value wisdom. Wisdom is at 385. Wise people tend to be benign. They're safe to be with— as safe as Koko. Humane, happy, and sensible. They're sometimes called "the salt of the earth."

There are various energy fields or chakra systems, as I'm sure you're aware. One collection of energy is at the lower mind. The lower mind is at 155. There's another collection of energy that we call the higher mind. They have two different sets of values.

What one setting considers to be valid and true and ethical, the other considers to be invalid and in fact immoral. The lower mind, then, is very interested in sensationalism, and is very gullible. It's interested in being smart and exploiting life. So, you might automatically think of the news. It likes to play off the sensational. It'll take some trivial little incident that is of no significance and give it major airtime. And something that really is of profound importance, and really threatens all of humanity, they give it only a glance—if that.

At 275 and up is the higher mind, and it is moving into thoughtfulness, balance, and sensitivity to what is appropriate and what is not appropriate. The higher mind tends to look for solutions, and tends to play off difficulties. So, there's a big payoff here. For 85 percent of the people in the world, their intellect is at this level. In America, only about 50 percent. About 50 percent of people would rather watch something gory and horrible and sensational than something that is inclusive of beauty. The power of consciousness is now recognized.

Einstein, who was a master of a linear dimension, calibrated at 499, and he refused to recognize the role of consciousness. He rejected its reality. He said, "I prefer to think there's a distinct, objective, linear reality out there." We've calibrated all these things to give you a scientific basis to understand how the phenomenal world occurs.

I always tell people, "Notice that everything is happening spontaneously." The limitation of the ego is it thinks there is a personal *I* as a cause, and based on the Newtonian principle, a *this* causing a *that*. In reality, there is no *this* causing any *that*. In fact, that phenomenon is not a possibility, because evolution and creation are one and the same thing. So, what you see is the emergence of potentiality as a consequence of evolution.

The limitation of the ego is it thinks there is a personal *I* as a cause, and based on the Newtonian principle, a *this* causing a *that*. In reality, there is no *this* causing any *that*. In fact, that phenomenon is not a possibility, because evolution and creation are one and the same thing.

TRANSCENDING THE MIND AND THE LINEAR DOMAIN

The reason for religious conflict is a lack of comprehension of the nature of divinity itself. It sees a God who starts here, and then one day creates all there is, and disappears. And after you die, you face him and greet him on judgment day. I don't know where he goes in the meantime, but he goes someplace. It's because the mind doesn't comprehend infinity.

To transcend the mind, which is based on cause and effect, and the Newtonian paradigm in science, you have to shift to a higher awareness. Stop projecting the idea of causality into the world. There is no causality in the world—none whatsoever. All that you perceive, and prove, and think is so out there is from your head, projected onto the world. Within the world, there is no causality. There is sequence. Sequence is not in the world either. Sequence means you perceived it sequentially. Therefore, you project that it must be in the world. It's your *perception* that's sequential.

How do things come about? The quickest way to enlightenment is to focus and notice that everything is, first of all, absolutely perfect. Everything is exquisite, perfect, and beautiful as it is, and things come about as a result of potentiality actualizing. Potentiality actualizes as a perceivable reality. So what you're witnessing, always, is the emergence of potentiality. The emergence of potentiality is for this arm to rise. It does it by itself. You think there's a you causing it, but you don't have anything to do with it. It rose itself, spontaneously.

All that's occurring spontaneously is due to the emergence of potentiality as actuality, when conditions are favorable. That's nonlinear dynamics, when conditions are favorable. So, the conditions also have to be favorable. You don't make the flower grow. I never saw anybody that made a flower grow. Did you ever meet anybody that made a flower grow? Thank you, God. When you plant something, you're taking advantage of what I just got through explaining. All you're doing is adding conditions that are favorable, such as sunlight, water, and fertilizer. But the potentiality is *within* the seed. It actualizes within the phenomenal world, not as causality. You can't *force* the flower to bloom.

We need to get rid of the idea of imperfection, because here, it has the potential to become a rose. The rose is half unfolded. You're going to tell me that's a bad rose? A defective rose? That something's wrong with the rose? No. You see, what happens is the potentiality actualizes, and it opens, and becomes actualized to your perception. Nothing is causing it to do that. You can't force a rose to do anything. It does it of its own accord, because it has, innate within its essence, the potentiality to manifest that way within the linear domain. All you're seeing is phenomena within the linear domain.

The energy of life is nonlinear, non-definable. And so, what I'm working on now is to resolve a dilemma of the Scopes Trial, which has to do with the argument of whether reality is limited to the linear—or does reality go on to include the nonlinear? The reasons the Scopes Trial couldn't be resolved is because they were talking about two different paradigms. The levels of consciousness go from, let's say, one to 1,000. Science is within the 400s, and spiritual reality starts from 500 and up. They are two different paradigms. So you can't resolve oil and water, because they're two different paradigms. Science can neither prove nor disprove spiritual reality, nor vice versa. It's a different paradigm.

What I'm trying to do is create a paradigm that includes both, which shows that you're just moving from one paradigm to another. This would be inclusive of both science and religion. You see, they're both true, and both 100 percent true *within* their own paradigms. So, it's really ignorance on the two sides to expect each other to agree, since they are each living from different paradigms of reality.

HIGHER LEVELS OF CONSCIOUSNESS

We went on to study various religions, and calibrate the levels of movies, books, television shows—everything represents a greater or a lesser degree of spiritual energy. The greater the spiritual orientation and the alignment with truth, the higher the calibration.

And so, we have this calibrated scale of consciousness, the greatest usefulness of which is really to say *yes* or *not yes*. So, you would say, "This spiritual teacher is integrous and useful for my life." And you get a yes or a not yes. Or you might say, "It's too soon. Maybe I should wait with this one." And it'll say yes or not yes. One can use it for guidance, and spiritual students who are really committed to transcending the ego and reaching the higher spiritual states have found it quite useful.

That state we call enlightenment occurs at a level calibrated at 600. When a person goes into 600, they go into the levels of love. First conditional love, then unconditional love. Then many become interested in spiritual pathways and meditation and spiritual techniques, and they begin to pursue them with greater and greater dedication. As they do, they begin to experience life in a transformative, completely different context.

In the high 500s, which are quite amazing, one is overcome by the sheer beauty of everything. The only reality that exists is love. There's only love, and all you see is love. All you experience is love and beauty. Love, beauty, and harmony, and the miraculous begin to happen spontaneously, and eventually they become continuous.

A lot of people who've done *A Course in Miracles* go into that transformative state. You drive into the city, and you think of a parking space, and as you get there, there's a parking space waiting right in front of you. In fact, it's the one and only parking space, and just as you pull up, a car pulls out and you pull in. When this first begins to happen, you sort of remark about it. After a while, you begin to experience that that's the way life is. It's the continuous miraculous. The miraculous is ongoing and continuous.

In this state, everybody becomes stunningly beautiful and handsome. You are in love. This isn't about falling in love. You are in love with everything and everyone, all the time. And you can only see the beauty and perfection of everything.

And then, the state may reach, in the very high 500s, ecstasy. One can start going into states of indescribable ecstasy, like the opening of a brilliance within one's consciousness. The ecstasy is continuous. At that point, you can't function in the world anymore—the ecstasy, as Ramakrishna described it. I remember going through it myself. Forget about functioning in the world. You can dance. You can dance in an expression of exquisite ecstasy at the joy of one's existence. But you cannot function.

And then, one has to surrender that to God. So each step along the way of the levels of consciousness is surrendering whatever is presenting itself to God. Finally, even in the state of ecstasy, one has to surrender the state of ecstasy to God. And then one hits level 600, which is a state of infinite silence, bliss, and a profound peace beyond all understanding. The peace of God is beyond psychological peace or emotional peace. It's a different dimension. And in that state, you don't have to eat, breathe, or function. One blisses out, outside of time. *Satchitananda* it's called, classically.

And if things are favorable, the body will eventually get fed, move up and walk around, and survive. If the conditions are not favorable to that circumstance, which frankly is irrelevant, then the body just topples over eventually. So about 50 percent of the people who go into a latent state frankly, leave. The one awareness that is quite obvious in that state is that you have permission to leave. You can leave right now, in fact. You can stop reading. You have permission.

So, what's going to keep the body going? Well, you see, there are no needs and no wants. Everything is complete and total. The bliss of the state is that everything is complete. So, from that moment on, if the body survives, you don't ever really need anything anymore. People ask, "What do you want?" I don't want anything. "What do you need?" Well, I don't *need* anything. Certain things would be nice, but I don't *need* them.

And so, one is then independent of the world. What the world says or does is really quite irrelevant. At that point, it's impossible to function in that state. What happens, if you survive, is most people leave. They pack up everything, say good-bye, and leave. This is what I did. I left the biggest practice in the country and a very elite lifestyle, and I drove to a small town. In the refrigerator, there'd be a banana, two Pepsis, and a piece of cheese, and that was fine. What more do you need?

Chapter 3

SPIRITUAL
CONSCIOUSNESS

---

*Now that you have a clearer understanding of how to cal-
ibrate spiritual truth and the Map of Consciousness, you are
ready to begin elevating your level of spiritual consciousness to
its highest potential.*

*In this chapter, Dr. Hawkins will give you several ideas for
doing just that. They include relinquishing the quest for perfection;
following evolved spiritual values rather than dogmatic religious
doctrines; and being grateful, introspective, and compassionate.*

You are not limited by this world, or even definable, measur-
able, and visible. By looking at the levels of consciousness on
the chart, you can tell what your spiritual worth is.

You want to transcend the world—that is, to be in it, but not of
it, not limited by it. To be limited by it is to buy all of its programs.
To buy all of its programs, you're going to have to run around and
buy everything that's for sale, because if you're successful, you'll
have new carpets and you'll have a new house. You can't possibly
meet all the definitions of "making it" in this world: you should
have more friends, you should be handsome, or you should be six
feet tall.

There's always something you can find fault with when it comes to yourself; you'll never be satisfied. The thing is to be happy with what you are at the moment, and also see that you're an evolving human being. Therefore, you don't have to be perfect because you're not required to be perfect. You're only expected to make the best possible use you can of the advantages here, to learn and to grow and to support others, and to be loving and forgiving. And you're doing all you can do as a human being.

BECOMING A SPIRITUAL SEEKER

There are fewer religionists and more spiritually evolved people—more people who call themselves spiritual rather than religious. It's because of the downside of religion, historically. Every religion has had historical events that would disqualify it hypothetically. *How can they have made such a mistake? How can I believe a church that believed in that, or made that mistake?* But what goes on is people will call themselves spiritual; that's the most common pattern in today's world. They begin to follow spiritual values and they learn from spiritual teachers, alive or historical.

Most spiritual teachers have considerable followings of people who are interested in evolving and growing, maturing spiritually in their levels of consciousness. And they may stay there with one teacher, or they may go to a number of teachers. There was a period of time of being a spiritual seeker, where you went to lots of lectures by all different kinds of spiritual teachers. Each one has something valuable that you can pick up from them: techniques or ways of looking at things, or a blind spot that you weren't aware you had until you hear a lecture on it.

So, you seek—you become a spiritual seeker. In a way, spiritual really means seeking. See, with religion, you found the answer. That's this church and this denomination, and that's the answer. Now you just have to perfect how you apply it to yourself. The spiritual person who says, "I'm spiritual, but not religious," usually becomes a seeker. They go to various lectures, and they attend meetings and retreats. And they listen to all the different teachers and learn something from each one. Each spiritual teacher has something. And what they have may be nonverbal—the subtle enthusiasm they have for certain concepts, et cetera.

And the seeker picks up that enthusiasm. So each teacher has something to share and something that can be learned. Most of my own audiences listen to a number of different speakers. Each of these teachers may be suitable at various periods of your life. There are certain times when going on spiritual retreats is extremely valuable, and then there are other times when that's just a way of avoiding the responsibilities of life. You really had a lot you should have done at home this weekend and instead, you went on a retreat to Camp Baba. When you get home, the lawn still hasn't been mowed. The kids are still crying. You didn't help the kids with their homework. When you're running away, you're really doing it for an advantage. Most of these spiritual things serve a purpose at certain periods of your life. I've noticed most people change their pattern as they go through life, if they're going to evolve. Other people just develop a perfect pattern and stay with that; they stay with that for a lifetime.

• • •

To just be grateful that you're interested in the spiritual dimension at all—that's already something to be grateful for. I mean, how many people lead a blind life? They calibrate at 192 when they come onto the planet, and when they leave, they calibrate at 192. No change. So they really blew a whole lifetime, just doing the same self-centered, greedy things all the time. The Buddha said, "Rare it is to be born a human, rarer still it is to have heard of enlightenment, and rarest of all it is to have heard of enlightenment and dedicate oneself to its pursuit." That's the rarest of all. So to be dedicated to the searching for the truth, is the rarest of all possible gifts.

As a human, you can undo negative karma and gain positive karma. And if you use these lifetimes on earth wisely, you can reach enlightenment. So be grateful that one is a human and that one has heard of the truth.

• • •

Be introspective; you can't walk around naively oblivious of who you are and how you come across to people. So you need a certain degree of self-awareness and the capacity for self-criticalness—to be able to see your upside, your downside, and your limitations; accept the reality of your personality where it is; and be introspective and reflective. Somebody else will suggest something, and you say, "Well, I have to reflect on that." It means you're going to hold it in mind and various facets begin to reveal themselves. You forget all about it and then you have a peanut butter sandwich, and in the middle of the sandwich you realize other significances of it—how it affects your relationships with others, how it reflects the fulfillment of things you've held in mind, the implicit limitations of what you feel you would not be able to do, et cetera.

So significance and fulfillment, all these things become consequences of reflection. What's the saying? "The unexamined life is not worth living." We need to be conscious and aware. And many people are extremely oblivious to how they come across to others—unaware of major blind spots and repetitious behavior. They make the same mistake for decades. And you wonder, *Why haven't they gotten any feedback from the world, or reflected on that?* I think this has to do with the capacity to constantly learn to have an open mind, to be able to ask, and to do so with perspicacity. The capacity to discern and observe. And of course, one of the things about being a physician is you need *perspicacity.*

And over the years, I could always tell who was outside my office. I would hear the next patient coming across the floor to the office door, and I could already tell whether they were better or worse than last time. Somehow, the rate, the gait, the rhythm, their stance as they walked into the room already said a great deal about the person. So with perspicacity, you have to be able to witness the slightest alteration of things. There are people who are completely oblivious. They walk around in a dream state or something.

The interest in the evolution of one's own consciousness—how it's evolved over time, how it expressed itself in ancient times—is still present in today's world. There are people who are still mystics in this world, who speak from the Self. Curiosity leads to learning. That's how the little amoeba stays alive. It has to constantly search around and find something to eat or it's not going to be here. People do get addicted to the accumulation of knowledge for its own sake. And that's probably just a phase that people go through, and sooner or later, one begins to realize that it has to be put into actual practice and then just be intellectually conversant. That's just part of the evolution of one's spiritual awareness.

First you accumulate the information, then, you pursue the information to experience for yourself the truth of it. People often start out with intellectual curiosity, and they'll buy just about any and every book they can on spirituality. I went through that phase myself. I had a whole wall of books on everything you can think about: pseudo spirituality, true spiritualty, psychic readings, people on the other side, channelings, and God knows what else. And then discernment arose over the years. So, there's a curiosity—sort of a wide-eyed amazement that there are realms that you weren't even aware of. You can go through formal schooling and never be aware that there's anything other than the logical, linear under the concrete. And suddenly you become aware that there are whole dimensions.

SURRENDERING THE SMALL SELF

The personal will is trying to accomplish something as a very specific goal. It usually has to do with gain or dominance or control in some way. The spiritual world is more in the field of surrender. Now the personal will is only as strong as one's level of consciousness. So sometimes people will want to accomplish something by personal will, and that would require much more power than the personal will. Let's say you live at consciousness level 190, and now through personal will, you're going to try to overcome a certain thing, but you don't have enough power at consciousness level 190. When you get up to consciousness level 500 or so, now you would have the power to overcome it, but you haven't got enough horsepower in the engine to do it at that level. Therefore, aligning yourself with a more powerful field is what people do.

For example, let's look at addiction. While the addiction may take you all the way down to consciousness 90, to surrender to God's will is something that you don't have the strength to do yourself. A person takes you to an AA meeting, which calibrates at 540. At the consciousness level of 540, the person says, "Well, you could let go of the addiction if you wanted to." And suddenly it dawns on you, that's true. It isn't *could you*, it's *would you*. When people have trouble making spiritual decisions, here's another example I give them. Somebody says, "I can't possibly forgive my ex-brother-in-law for what he did to me." And I'll say, "Now, if I have a .45 loaded next to your temple, and if you don't forgive him, I'm going to blow your brains out. Could you forgive him?"

"Oh yes, I could." So, I say, "Well, that clearly differentiates the *could* from *would*." And mostly what people think is *could*, is just that they *wouldn't*. They're unwilling to do it. If you're willing to forgive anybody, you can forgive anybody for anything. It's the will. So surrendering the will to God is important; you see, divine will calibrates extremely high, at about 850. Your personal will, near 190, is something different. When you surrender your will to God, now you can accomplish the *miraculous*. It isn't you that accomplishes it—you've surrendered the small self to the large Self. The large Self counts on the will of God to accomplish its goals, and therefore is capable of performing the miraculous. And when you get to a certain level of consciousness, the miraculous becomes continuous. What people think is miraculous is really just our innocence.

When you get to a certain level—around 570 or 580—the miraculous becomes ordinary. You hold the thing in mind and it manifests, and you don't go: "Oh, isn't that amazing?" That's the way it all happens. It all unfolds based on how it's being held in mind. And it's because the Self, with the capital *S*, can accomplish what the small self cannot do, even though its life depends on it. People try and they actually die in the attempt. They do not have the power. Because force results in counter force, and surrender pulls you in a powerful context. When you say, "God, I of myself, am unable to do a certain thing, and I ask you if it is your will, that it be accomplished," and then you surrender it, at that point, you really surrender it. You don't keep insisting that God do it or not do it.

At that point, you *relinquish* the personal will. And that which you thought was going to be impossible, now comes about in the most miraculous and unbelievable way. And if you put a string of miraculous experiences together, a skeptic would have a hard time trying to figure out how best to explain such a number of phenomena. And when the phase of the siddhis appears, the miraculous is numberless and almost continuous. One would wonder how to explain this from the viewpoint of pedestrian logic, and the simplicity of scientific thinking. How is it that in the entire parking paradox of New York City, the only parking space suddenly opens up just as you drive up?

Well, that's the way it was for years. What's the probability of that? Practically nothing. That was followed by something else. We followed one phenomenon after another in which its statistical probability is nil. And when we put them together—the nil plus nil plus nil, plus nil—we wonder how to explain this phenomena.

You might not know where you're going and start driving to a strange town, and pull up right exactly to the place you wanted to go—because all you did is hold it in mind. I used to do that all the time: just held in mind Florida, all around lakes that I didn't know, one lake from another. I automatically drove exactly where I wanted to go, with no map and no knowledge of the territory.

So that's just one example, but those things are continuous. There's a phase where it goes on for years, the unfolding of everything is continuous. You need a pair of pliers, so you look out the window of the truck and not only is there a pair of pliers laying there by the road, but they're a *brand-new* pair of pliers. Laying there within an arm's reach—they're brand new. And you don't even say "wow" anymore, because this is the way life has become. You're hungry, and around the next turn there's a hamburger joint. There you are. Life becomes one hamburger joint after another.

BECOMING THE WITNESS

It's very easy to see that everything is happening spontaneously, that even your thinkingness is happening all on its own. You think that you're deciding what you're going to think, but you're not, so you get detached from your own thinkingness, the same as the world. You see that the world around you is moving without your help. All these people are managing to survive without you helping them to be here, and move, and talk. And so what you do is you get detached and you begin to become the witness. To become the witness is not a difficult step; it's only a matter of letting go of the narcissistic self-indulgence of thinking that there's an *I* causing things. Nothing is causing anything. There are no causes in the world.

There are only consequences. And so what you do is you let go of identifying with the linear, and you realize that your reality is nonlinear. You see that which is witnessing, and then behind that which is witnessing, that which is aware that you're witnessing— and already you've removed yourself from out there and from the individual, personal I, and from the guilt and anxiety of being the cause of all that happens. You've moved into the condition of humility. With profound humility, you'll see that you're not the cause of anything, which is welcome news because that means you're also not guilty of anything. Something happens, and you say, "I don't know, the mind did it. The mind did it. I can't help it, the mind did it!"

So, to become the witness then, you become aware of the spontaneity of evolution, and you begin to witness. All phenomena are the evolution of creation. Creation has a source, but no cause; it has no beginning, and it has no end. You witness the unfoldment of creation. There is no problem with creation because it's what you're witnessing. The fact that it's all happening spontaneously is not difficult to see. This observation escapes about 99 percent of mankind.

At least 99 percent of humanity is completely unaware of this. And we're not counting on widespread acceptance that you are the context rather than the content. You are that from which awareness radiates and out of which consciousness arises. The source is consciousness itself. The light of God is consciousness. The light of God is your own consciousness. And as you let go of misidentifying with that which you are not, it becomes stunningly apparent.

THE SOUND OF GOD IS SILENCE

Silence calibrates at 1,000. The sound of God is silence. To have sound, you have to have linearity; you have to have that which is sound and that which is not sound, and then you have to give a configuration to the sound. Therefore, mantras and other things like saying "om" will take you to a certain level. And beyond that, you become aware of the silence *behind* the sound. And so, the purpose of the sound is to take you to the silence. That's why repeating a mantra can sometimes really just lead to an altered state of consciousness and the high feeling that you get disappears when you stop the mantra.

The sound of God is silence.

Mantras have limited usages. They can assist at certain points, but you can't live your whole life as a mantra. You can, however, live your whole life as a prayer, because a prayer is a verbalization of a nonlinear intentionality, a prayer to make your life a prayer to become that—and that which you are speaks louder than what you say. Essence speaks louder than perception. The levels of consciousness don't say that you're better than others. It's not a matter of better, but because of our status-oriented society, we say it's better. It's not better—it's different. And very often, to be in a different state of consciousness that is not appropriate to where you are can be a hindrance.

To be blissed-out when you're driving is not so great. You have to pull over. So, you have to sort of be in what's appropriate to the situation. That begins to adjust itself automatically. It is true that if you suddenly advance to a higher state, you may be quite incapacitated, so it's good to have spiritual friends, and hang out with spiritual people and let them know that you're seriously on a spiritual path.

LIFTING THE CONSCIOUSNESS LEVEL OF MANKIND

People think it's what you do or what you say or how you behave that matters. No, it's the *consequence* of that which you are. So that which you are, if you sit alone in a cave, is influencing the consciousness level of mankind. Even if you sit alone in a cave, it radiates out as an energy. So each one's contribution raises the level of the sea. People will ask me, "What can I do to help the world?" The best thing you can do is become the fulfillment of your own potential, because each inch that the sea rises lifts all the ships afloat. Now, nobody has enough strength in and of himself to lift a ship, but everybody is contributing.

So when everyone aligns themselves with spiritual integrity, to be as unconditionally loving as possible, then we all lift the level of the sea. And by lifting the level of the sea, we lift everyone on it. So we do what we can to lift the level of consciousness of mankind. And that influence then will have its influence.

The more aligned you are with spiritual reality, integrity, truth, and the universal love, the more profoundly you're effecting the world without having to do anything. Of course, doing good things works. There's nothing wrong with that. I'm not saying that. But in and of itself, that which you are and have become is what is truly influencing the world.

The more aligned you are with spiritual reality, integrity, truth, and the universal love, the more profoundly you're effecting the world without having to do anything.

• • •

The willingness to surrender how you see things, then, begins to transform how you see and experience life. Instead of being angry and condemning others, you see that people cannot help being the way they are. Let's say there are these teenagers throwing rocks at each other and provoking the police into attacking them. You begin to see they can't help themselves. As you really go into great depth, you begin to discern the basic innocence of human consciousness. The consciousness itself is like the hardware of a computer, and the ego is like the software. The consciousness itself is unable to tell truth from falsehood. It cannot tell whether it's being programmed, like the Nazis did with the Nazi youth, into falsehood, or whether it's truth.

So then you understand why Christ and Buddha said, "Forgive them for they know not what they do." The hardware of the computer is unaltered by the software. The consciousness of the youth is innocent. So those kids who threw rocks then are looked at with compassion. You can see that they have been abused somehow. You see their spiritual abuse. And because of the innocence of human consciousness, its inability to discern truth from falsehood, mankind is led down the path of falsehood.

We can think of the young people in Nazi Germany, being patriotic. It's like going to Boy Scout camp—they're around the campfires, singing songs and hiking and doing all this for their country, for their fatherland, for the Führer. How could they have believed anything other than that? If we'd been there, we would've been doing the same thing. You see the innocence. So we begin to see the basic innocence of human consciousness, and now it allows us to forgive everyone. You see that everybody's being run by the programs with which they've been programmed. I mean, what else could they think? People believe the media because television comes across so fast; they've already believed it before they've had a chance to even examine their questioning.

The mind gets programmed. And so you see on the one hand, the ego survives by juicing negativity; on the other hand, it can't help but do that. It can't help but be that which it is. And without the power of spiritual truth, frankly, it's unable to transcend itself. The value of spiritual truth is that without it, nobody would transcend the ego. It's because of the great avatars, it's because of the great power of spiritual truth, and those who have realized the reality, then there lies the source of their own existence. That creates the power of the field, and the power of the field is where people derive inspiration to then transcend their limitations.

We understand then that basically human consciousness is innocent—it doesn't know truth from falsehood. The reason I had to write the book *Power vs. Force* is because it staggered me, and I realized man has never had a chance to know truth from falsehood. The best man has been able to do is to follow the intellect and end up at a consciousness level of 460, which leaves you stuck right in the middle of the mind and its dualities, and therefore war and hatred and all are destined to go on and on and on—because without spiritual energy and truth to transcend it, the mind is hopelessly caught in its own web. And it gets paid off for getting so, as it goes round and round and round and ruminates—it gets a payoff. Therefore, it's self-propagating.

The ego unaided, without external spiritual truth, will forever go round and round chasing its own tail. Each person, as they do what they think is personal spiritual work, is actually influencing the entire field. The prevailing level of consciousness of mankind then progresses as a consequence of the collective spiritual effort of all of us. Every choice, every spiritual decision we make reverberates around the universe. Like it says in scripture, "Not one hair of your head goes uncounted." And we discovered with muscle testing that that is a fact. Anything anybody's ever done, thought, felt—every decision that's ever been made—is recorded forever in the field of consciousness.

People who say they don't believe in karma can do so as a belief system. But they would still have to explain how it is that all phenomena that have ever occurred throughout all of history are recorded forever. How do you explain that every entity that gets born on this planet already has a calibrated level of consciousness? Therefore, we did not arise out of nothingness, but out of somethingness. And what is that somethingness out of which we all arise into which we all return? That takes us out of the limitation of the timeframe of the present. And we begin to see an experienced life in a greater dimension and the spiritual realities that arise out of contemplating such things encourage our investigation into spiritual truth, which is the purpose of this kind of work.

I wanted to first present the whole panorama of consciousness—its evolution, its quality, its nature, and how it's been approached through science, reason, logic, philosophy, ethics, theology, and religion. How it has evolved in mankind, how it manifests itself and the part that it plays in everyday life. Force then requires energy, and it exhausts people. People can only exert force to a certain point, and then they begin to collapse. Power, on the other hand, does not exhaust itself. In fact, the more it's used, the more powerful it seems to be. For instance, if we experiment with forgiving people and being willing to love and love unconditionally, we find that that capacity grows.

In the beginning, it may seem difficult to love that which seems unlovable, but if we dedicate ourselves to that way of being in the world, if we dedicate ourselves to being that way in the world, then we find that it's easier and easier. We find that with force, the more you give away, the less you have. But with power, the more you give, the more you have. So the more loving a person is, the more loving their world becomes. We begin to experience the world of our own creation. Some people say, "You go to New York City, and they're all so cold and horrible there. I hate New York City; they're all mean." And another person goes to New York City and says, "My goodness, they were the most wonderful people—all the waitresses and cabdrivers were so neat . . . it's just an incredible place!" Well, it's because in the presence of love, we precipitate the emergence of love in other people. And when we're not loving, we tend to bring forth the negative side of their natures.

We find that with force, the more you give away, the less you have. But with power, the more you give, the more you have.

So all we're experiencing then is the kind of a world that we're precipitating. A virtual display of what we and ourselves have become.

• • •

The contrast between power and force is given dramatically by historical example of the British empire, vis-à-vis Mahatma Gandhi. Well, Mahatma Gandhi, as you know, was a Hindu ascetic. And if you calibrate Gandhi, he's over 700. At the time that he confronted the British empire, it was the greatest force the world had ever seen. It ruled one quarter of the world, a third of the planet and the seas.

And when I was growing up, it was still the great British empire upon by which the sun never set. Against that stood a little 90-pound Hindu, skin and bones—he confronted the great lion who ruled one-third of the planet. The interesting thing is that Mahatma Gandhi, by doing nothing—in fact, just *saying* he's going to stop eating, and if they didn't like it, he'd just starve to death—threw the world into a panic. And at 700 Gandhi stood there. Well, 700 is of course enormous power, extremely rare on the planet. He faced off against the British empire, which in its pridefulness and self-interest calibrated at 190.

And without firing one single shot Gandhi defeated the entire British empire and took it apart, and brought the end of colonialism. It was not only the British empire, but colonialism per se, that he defeated, and self-rule became the dominant political system in the world. What Gandhi really represents then is the influence of power. Power doesn't *cause* things; force can be said to cause things within the Newtonian paradigm. Power *influences* things.

Now, you know that a quark is going to rise depending on the density of the medium that it finds itself in. So by prayer, by spiritual evolution, what happens then is that mankind creates a very powerful field, this field, this spiritual reality, which then begins to lift and effect all of mankind. It effects the whole paradigm of reality and values. So as I mentioned before, integrity is now becoming a predominant value in our society; it's being talked about constantly in the media. We have a whole new value system. Now, that was not brought about by the mechanism of force. Nobody forced the media to begin valuing integrity, but integrity emerged as a social value. Not as a spiritual value, but as a social value.

We all live by our own principles. Spiritual growth then means, What principles do we live by? And as we grow and mature, we choose different principles. Some people live by the principle of "Always be right—never give the sucker a break." People come out and state what their principles are. Sometimes they seem quite outlandish, but you could say they're integrous to the degree that they live by them. To the degree that they live by them, they are living by what they're committed to. So I respect what people say they're committed to, and I think to the degree they live by that, then they're being virtuous by their own definition. So the calibrated level of consciousness, to some degree, then reflects the degree to which we live by our own stated spiritual choice.

You might say karma or spiritual destiny, the calibrated level of consciousness, then, is the consequence of spiritual freedom of choice. So we have freedom of choice at every moment, but this freedom of choice seems to be obscure. We seem to be run by programs. And one reason that we try to transcend the ego is because we don't want to be at the effect of the ego. We would like the mind to stop long enough for us to deliberate and make a choice. And so often we do a thing quickly and we regret it later, and sort of get a feeling of resentment, thinking, *Gee, I didn't really have a moment to really think about that.*

Our spiritual choices, then, tend to determine which direction we choose when the moment arises. If it wasn't for the silence of consciousness, you would not be able to know what you're thinking. It's because of the silence of the forest that you can hear sound. It's because the mind is silent that you can hear or see or picture what you're thinking. Therefore, the content of the mind must be going on in the space of no mind, which is a classical term, meaning thoughtless, formless consciousness, upon which thoughts reflect themselves. So, we withdraw our investment and preoccupation and identification with the content of thinking and begin to see that *we're* the space in which thinking can occur.

The value of meditation, then, is that it focuses us so that we withdraw our investment in identification with the content of thought to the space in which the thought is occurring. We begin to see that there is a *witness* to the thinking. There is an awareness to the witness, and there's a substrate that underlies all of it that is beyond time, beyond dimension, and that it is independent of personal identification. And the identification then with consciousness itself lifts us out of the identification of our reality as either the body or the mind or the thoughts or the feelings, and takes us to a greater dimension.

As we move into that greater dimension, then we confirm the spiritual reality, which underlies our existence. People become involved in spiritual work on a practical level. They want to know, "How can I forgive my enemies when I hate them so much after all they've done to me? How can I feel hope when I'm really depressed? How can I get rid of fear when I'm scared all the time?" It starts out on a very practical level. Other people will start out from a different level. They start out through inspiration. They will hear an inspirational speaker and get uplifted.

One can start from curiosity; one can start from sort of a spontaneous evolution within one's own consciousness. I think spiritually evolved people inspire others outside of their awareness. Because they influence the field, people who would have ordinarily not been interested in spirituality suddenly become curious—not through any inner prompting, but as a consequence of the field. So if you're around people who are more spiritually evolved, you may find your own interest in it spontaneously becoming more intense. It's not through any deliberate decision-making, but just because it's more interesting—like how when you're around people who are into sports, you tend to listen more and be more interested in that.

When people have some kind of disaster in their life—and we hear it all the time about an illness or drugs or alcohol or criminality or grief or loss—they want to know what they can do about it. The willingness to surrender life to God, of course, is one of the most profound spiritual tools. People ask, "What spiritual tools are the most powerful?" I would say, humility, the willingness to surrender life—to let go of wanting to control it, to let go of wanting to change it—the willingness to surrender how you see things to God (or to some higher spiritual principle, because God is not a reality. It's just a word to most people).

For most people, God is a hoped-for reality, but not an experiential reality until they become more spiritually advanced and begin to experience the presence of the field itself and intuit its enormous power. Then they revere God, because they respect the infinite power that they begin to intuit. What we can do on a practical level, then, is become the best person we can become. I'd say to become kind toward all of life in all of its expressions, no matter what. And that includes oneself: to be willing to forgive oneself, to see the limitation of human consciousness.

I always feel that the more educated you are about the quality of consciousness, the nature of consciousness, the easier it is to follow spiritual principles. If you understand that human consciousness is intrinsically innocent and cannot control that which it is programmed by, because it can't tell truth from falsehood, you begin to feel compassion automatically.

Chapter 4

OBSTACLES TO
SPIRITUAL GROWTH

Oftentimes, the harder one tries to pursue a spiritual path, the more they can feel like they are getting nowhere, continually pulled down by the cares of this world or the feeling of desolation and abandonment by the divine. In this important chapter, Dr. Hawkins discusses these obstacles to spiritual growth so that you can identify them, overcome or avoid them, and get back on the spiritual path. Dr. Hawkins begins by discussing how following false spiritual teachers who promise to unveil unknown spiritual secrets can be one of the greatest obstacles to true spiritual wisdom.

There's a great deal of spiritual fiction out there. In fact, the best-selling spiritual books are all fiction. *The DaVinci Code*, for example. There are all kinds of psychics who tell all kinds of stories about the end of the world or the code of God hidden in your genes. That which is spiritual truth is not invisible nor is it encoded. It's starkly wide open. There would be no point to hide the secrets. What kind of secrets are you talking about? There are no secrets to hide.

Spiritual truth is transparent. For that which is veiled, mysterious, cloaked, you have to pay money. "Mystical secret of the ancients! Give me $500! I will whisper the secret of life into your ears!" And then you say this mantra at the same time, "Oom boom boomy boom. Oom boom boomy boom." You can see the profit motive. Spiritual truth has nothing to gain by its promulgation. It doesn't even care if you agree with it or not. Anybody can repudiate anything I say, and it's certainly their option. I have no quarrel with it. There are no qualifications; you don't have to be or prove anything. You don't have to pay anything. You don't have to sign anything. You don't have to justify. You don't have to prove that you have any right or claim.

Spiritual truth is transparent.

A true spiritual teacher *frees* you and so-called charlatans try to bind you. They try to own you, control you, tell you what to do. Spiritual truth is freely given. It's not provisional to conditions or who believes it or who doesn't believe it—or whether it's provable or not provable, because what the world considers provable is not provable. It's not aligned with any particular thing. It doesn't have to exist here or there or be on a mountaintop—as if we can only have a holy order on top of a mountain at 6,000 feet.

RELIGIONISM AND THE DANGERS OF A NARCISSISTIC EGO

A lot of people think they're religious and really what they're practicing is *religionism*. The main problem with religion now is we deify the religion rather than God. The printed word or the teaching of a teacher now transcends divinity itself. You find you're not worshiping God; you find that people worship the religion rather than the *truth of the religion*. In the name of the religion, you have the inquisition. Religionism then eventually becomes its own opposite.

We know if you add *-ism* to the end of any area of knowledge, that it automatically drops to 190. Now it becomes positionalized with narcissistic gain. So, you have to impose environmentalism. You have to impose liberalism. You have to impose conservativism. The minute it's an ism—militarism or antimilitarism—it becomes a crusade, and everybody wants to get on the bandwagon and get on TV and hold up a placard. The vanity of the narcissistic ego is unlimited.

• • •

Through education, you get what the limitations of the ego are, and that gives you a certain degree of humility to begin with. You realize that you're lucky to have any idea what reality is in the first place, because the ego is so intent on displacing reality with its own perceptions and projecting them onto the world that it's almost impossible to see the reality of the world, because so much is projection. The media, first of all, by what they select have already prejudiced you. They say, "Oh, this is important; that's why it's on the evening news." Things that are profoundly more important are *never* on the evening news. Only the trivial is on the evening news. The profoundly important would not be of interest to people.

How did the great shakers and makers of this world arrive at their conclusions and execute them? That would be worth looking at instead of the latest titillations and silly amusements we see. How do the great people think, and why do they arrive at the conclusions they arrive at, and how can that be contextualized so that we can understand it? How to understand the world that we see would be far more interesting, but many people are not that interested in looking past appearance. I'm always interested in what the essence of a thing is. I know what the appearance is. I can flick on the news and see it for myself. But what is the essence of that? Is it naivete? Very often, it is.

Spiritual humility is an attitude I have myself. My mind, in and of itself, is not really capable of discerning the ultimate truth. That's why the great avatars came to reveal to us that which is unknowable. And to be grateful all the time is an attitude of humility. To be grateful that you're interested in spirituality, you say, "I'm grateful I'm even interested in the subject. I'm grateful that I've come across good teachers along the way. I'm grateful for the life experiences that have come about, that have revealed truths to me."

So you must understand that humility is a positionality. It's where you stand back and you're sort of saying, "I have myself been unable to fully comprehend it." And you're constantly asking for revelation. So your position with God is like a mudra. Your position with God is like yin. It's when you stand back and you say, "To thee, oh Lord, I surrender, and I ask for your will in the matter." And then you surrender to what appears to be most aligned with divinity.

• • •

All negative feelings are linked with each other. You want something because you feel unfulfilled. So if something gets in the way, now you get angry. Now you get frustrated, and you realize that if you get it, now you're going to be prideful. But if you're prideful in your ownership, now you have to fear that somebody will take it away from you or that you won't get it. And then you get puffed up if you do have it. So one thing leads to another. Your anger is that somebody is interfering. Negative feelings are all based on the same delusion. And the delusion is that the source of happiness is something outside of yourself.

When I get that title, when I get that car, when I get that job, when I get that income, when I get that—there's always a *get*—when I get that relationship, when I get that recognition, when I get on the TV program, when I get on the nightly news, I'll be somebody. It's always a gettingness. If anything stands in your way to getting this, now you hate it and you're angry at it, and you want to destroy it. When you see that one thing leads to another, then if you don't achieve it, you feel guilt and self-blame and you feel worthless. Now you feel depressed.

All the negative feelings are based on the assumption that what you need is outside of yourself. You see yourself as incomplete. And once I'm famous, once I'm educated, once I'm older, once I'm richer, once I'm . . . then I'll be happy. No matter what you say, it always puts fulfillment off in the future. So you're always coming from incomplete to incomplete, because *you're* incomplete. But then when you get what you want, there's always one better. I knew many super rich people back East. And they always had the saying: No matter how big your yacht is, a bigger one will dock next to you.

It's an endless race, and it was very comical to see it. And of course, people who are really quite wealthy and have been for some time, live very simple lives save for public events and parties.

I knew lots of multimillionaires, and very often they would inherit a big estate—40 acres with a huge castle of a house and all these buildings—and when I went to visit them, they actually lived in one of the servant's houses. There's a little house out there, and that's where they lived. The richest people in America! I used to live next door to one, and he had a third story on his house. And I said, "What's up there?" He said, "I don't know, I've never been up there." They would usually stay put in two or three rooms in this giant house, the family estate, and there'd be a kitchen, a sitting room, and a bedroom. And that's where they lived 99 percent of the time, except when their great-niece was there and having a birthday party. And then they would have a party on the lawn, but they lived all the time in just a little corner of the house.

What are you going to do on the third floor with 5,000 feet of magnificent furniture and you? You and 5,000 feet of antique, beautiful furniture with a wonderful view . . . once you have looked out the window and seen the beautiful view, now what are you going to do? You go back downstairs to the kitchen and watch the TV, put your feet up, and put some wood in the stove, the same as the servants do. It's comical.

PARANORMAL REALMS AND DIMENSIONS

Straight and narrow is the path. You can spend quite a few lifetimes wandering through the fantasy world of psychics and channelers and people like this, the world of tarot cards and tea leaf readings. They are usually a dead end. Some entity on the other side tells you about a whole other dimension. Next thing you know, you're all involved in that dimension. A lot of them have gods with a weird name and various hierarchies. And a lot of times, for additional money, they will move you up to a different, higher level of anarchy. For another $5,000, they'll introduce you to master so-and-so on a different level, who will now give you some magical powers.

The whole thing is seductive. What's being seduced is the innocent curiosity of the child. For $5,000, they'll raise your level of consciousness a hundred points an hour. For $50,000, they guarantee you'll be enlightened in six weeks. I suppose people like to send them money because they're still there. When you first realize that there's something other than just logic in the phenomenal world, the child in you goes, "Oh, wow."

I'm not saying the paranormal doesn't exist, but scripture says not to go there. Why? Because you're dealing in other realms, and you have no education or sophistication or awareness of the rules and the laws of those realms.

The angels fear to tread there. Why wouldn't you? It's morbid curiosity. You want to check out hell? You're not going to check out hell without getting burned. I advise people, don't go there. Don't be tempted by the drama of it. If you got to climb the highest mountain, make note of the fact that 176 people have died there already doing it. You can do the same thing. You can go out of body and visit other dimensions. You are not equipped to go there. You don't know anything about who's who there, and you're an innocent victim the minute you arrive. Tarot cards, Ouija boards, psychic readings, throwing runes are all forms of magic. The child in us is entranced by the magic.

I tell people not to try to calibrate low energies. You'll get attracted to that which is evil and demonic, and start trying to calibrate it, because your pendulum is going to get hit by that energy. And one of your energy fields and chakras can get reversed, by the way. Don't play around with it. The pendulum is not a game, and as with any kind of divination, it shouldn't be done for the sport.

Many people play with divination and we never hear from them again. I don't recommend it to people because it means they have to have some curiosity that is so hypothetical, it has nothing to do with their own spiritual destination. In other words, you're just asking out of idle curiosity. And often you're playing with very negative energies when you're doing that. You're trying to flirt with the negative and think you won't get burned. That's not going to happen. I know a lot of people who dealt with pendulums, started checking out other dimensions, and they really blew up and even became psychotic.

Many of these psychics over time turn out to be false. There's one locally that does all the things that are so typical of a cult. He tells people how to live, gets them bonded to him, tells them about their sex life. He makes them turn all of their money over to him. And one thing about these cult leaders you'll notice is that sex is forbidden to all the followers, but not to the cult leader. Well, of course, he's entitled to go to bed with anybody he wishes to, and then cite some entity on the other side. The fallacy of the whole thing is so transparent to a sophisticated person, but the person who gets entrapped into it, their inner child gets brainwashed by all this mumbo jumbo. And of course, we look at Jonestown as an example and wonder, how could a thousand sane adults commit suicide all at the same time? How could that be?

Cults, you see, are dangerous because they have the capacity to brainwash people. A teacher should free you, not bind you. You should not be bound by the teacher. On the contrary, you should be *freed* by the teacher. You owe nothing to a teacher whatsoever, except to be polite and listen if you wish. You're not in bondage, you don't owe, you're not obligated. A true teacher doesn't try to control you or get you to turn over your financial assets to them. The other thing false teachers do is theatrics, by which I mean putting on great displays with fancy robes and entourages and great wonders, buildings and all, to impress you with their importance. The other thing they try to impress you with is the number of followers. They have 10 million followers in India or something like that.

I calibrate the guy with 10 million followers, and he comes out at 140. So, we're a bit like lemmings being led over the cliff. Adolf Hitler had 40 million adoring followers too, and he calibrated at 90 and almost destroyed Germany and most of Europe! The fact that somebody has lots of followers doesn't mean a single thing whatsoever. Plus, some teachers start out integrous, reach a high place, and then fall. That is another innocence that the innocent person doesn't realize; that he was calibrated 570, but he's now at 190.

I always teach students that sooner or later, you're going to become a teacher. And each of the levels of consciousness has its downside and its traps. Once you become a teacher, there's this seduction of being glamorized; of being idolized; of people saying that they love you; of sexual seduction; and of the attraction of money, fame, and power over many people. Therefore, many are the gurus who began to ascend the path and then crashed. Half a dozen or more on TV or the Internet. They were at a high place at one point.

I believe a teacher should teach students that when you reach a certain level of consciousness, these are the temptations that you will be presented with. Don't forget the Buddha was beset by demons. And people think, *Oh, they're going to come in the form of evil demons.* Except they're not going to come in the form of evil demons; they're going to come in the form of seductions, sweet adoringness: *Oh, master!*

So that's the dramatization. I'm not saying that there isn't a lot to it. Scripture says it doesn't invalidate the paranormal; it just says, "Don't go there." You can have a couple of readings and become entranced. And then suddenly their readings go off, and some of the readings suddenly go wrong. So all those things, they're only tentative. And they're only transitory spiritual fiction, because then the reality seems mundane and pedestrian as compared to the magical wonderment or the tarot card reading or whatever. I think it's the wrong direction. And here the error is to fall for the seduction; that it is a quality or a power of your personal self, which it is not. The phenomena happen of their own accord. There is no personal self calling them.

We have witnessed miracles many times. And the trap is to think that *you* are the one who brought about the miracle. There is no person doing any miracles. The potentiation occurs when a certain energy field arises. It only happens when all the conditions are appropriate, including karmic conditions. When the apple is ready, it falls from the tree. Now the apple doesn't cause itself to fall from the tree. There's the field of gravity. So within the spiritual aura of an advanced teacher, phenomena that are due to occur karmically and for many reasons may be facilitated, but there's no personal self "doing" a cause-and-effect miraculous cure. You *witnessed* phenomena happen. You are the witness of them. And one is aware that yes, the energy field could exhilarate a propensity, but that karmic propensity is within the person himself. And all one did was facilitate it.

For example, a person who is very sick and disabled will sit down next to you, and then you can feel this energy move over in their domain, and then they'll get up and walk away. Well, you're aware it wasn't *you* that removed the illness, it was the energy, the Kundalini energy. Because of previous spiritual work that brought about an inner honesty and awareness, you just witnessed the phenomenon. It was the unfolding of potentiality emerging as a consequence of the energy fields surrounding it, which potentialized it. The Kundalini energy, by virtue of its own nature, is what is transformative and accomplishes the miraculous, not the personal you.

Everybody needs a teacher to warn them of this. Miracle workers are a dime a dozen. When the miracle came on, it was a phenomenon. Then the personal self took credit for that. Then the ego got exaggerated. Now they don't have that miraculous power anymore, but they don't want the world to know that, so they've learned how to fake it. And for one of the most famous gurus of recent times in India, the phenomena occurred spontaneously in the beginning. Then he claimed credit for it. Then he brought great throngs. They brought great money. Then he began to learn how to fake that which had before been autonomous. That's a very subtle thing. It's happened to more than one guru.

SPIRITUAL TRUTH

Now we're going to talk about spiritual truth. There are many false teachers in the world, and I was quite amazed when I discovered how many there were. I mean, lots who are world famous. Since you're putting your eternal soul in the hands of a teacher, you better know who that teacher is. I wouldn't be so careless. You're talking about your *eternal* soul, the karmic perpetuation throughout all of time, and you're going to put this in some flashy ad, go and get your aura read by Mr. So-and-So on the other side? Of course, you have to turn over all your property to him as well. You get a reading from master so-and-so through him, and it only costs you $5,000 for your granddaughter, except you don't have a granddaughter!

These gurus fell because their instructors did not instruct them of the downside. So in my lectures, we constantly go over: What is the downside of each level of consciousness? Where is the trap? People say, "I'm beyond that." You're not beyond that at all. From 850 and up, it's very difficult. And the Buddha acknowledged that; he said, "I felt like my bones are being broken," because the demons are looking for any weakness in your psyche. There are characteristics of spiritual truth that will carry you through if you know of them; you don't need a list of what they calibrate (though that's very handy). But if you know certain basics, it's more important to understand the basics. Truth is true at all times and places, independent of the culture, personalities, or circumstances.

Truth is always true, no matter what. So if we calibrate the Chartres cathedral, the calibration is the same no matter what. Truth is true at all times and places. It is not exclusionary; it's all inclusive, non-secretive, and non-sectarian. Nobody *owns* truth. One of the biggest traps is provisional love. There's energy of love—you become quite attractive to other people, and they will interpret it as love. People will fall in love with you all over the place. There was a period of time when I got propositioned a couple of times a day. And I didn't have a teacher to warn me. I knew the integrity of it was being tested. Many fall for that one. And then glamor—we weren't allowed to use the word *guru* in my book. Every time we would ask, it said, "No." The word has come to mean something different than what it originally meant, because it was being exploited. Wealth, fame, having lots of followers . . . all those things are temptations to the spiritual ego to consider yourself important. And you see how those spiritual egos throw it right back into a personal self, right away. The minute you think it's you, you just lost it.

Truth is always true, no matter what.

Truth is true everywhere; it excludes no one, is available and open to all. There are no secrets to be revealed, hidden, or sold— no magical formulas or mysteries. That is the truth. When we see an ancient secret being peddled, it's always for a price, and you know that you're being held up by a spiritual conman.

Truth to be truth is truth all the time: foreverness. And how could it be the exclusive property of someone? It's available and open to all. It has an integrity of purpose—there's nothing to gain or lose. It's nonsectarian; Truth is not the exposition of a limitation. Independent of opinion, truth is nonlinear. Therefore, it is not subject to the limitations of intellect or form. Truth is independent of opinion. Devoid of positionality, truth is not *anti*-anything. Why is that? Because truth has no opposite. You might say the opposite of truth is absence. Falsehood has no reality. There's truth and then there's the absence of truth, and we call the absence of truth, falsehood.

It's just like light and darkness. Light is either present or not present. There are no requirements or demands, no memberships, dues, fees, regulations, oaths, rules, or conditions. And it doesn't circularize everybody, asking for donations. It is non-controlling. Spiritual purity has no interest in the personal lives of the aspirants, in their clothing or dress, their style, their sex life, their economics, their family patterns, their lifestyle, or their dietary habits. It is free of force or intimidation. When people are threatened in their spiritual groups, or belong to the sect, there are recriminations if they try to get out of it. Sometimes punishment is quite severe. When there's truth, there's no force or intimidation, no brainwashing or adulation of the leaders, no training rituals. Watch out for training rituals—that's the call of brainwash by which you're indoctrinated.

If you know the truth, what do you need to be trained? Do not take any oaths. Do not pledge anything. "And if I fail to break these oaths, may such and such happen to me . . ." Never take such a vow. Truth is freedom; being free to come and go without persuasion, coercion, intimidation, or consequences. There is no hierarchy, and instead there is voluntary fulfillment of practical necessities and duties. Everyone I work with does what they do because that's what needs to be done.

If you do have a leader or people whom you honor, it's because of what one has become, rather than as a result of some title or trapping. You recognize truth when you see it. I respect all that exists because of the essence of that which they are, which I sense right away. Therefore, you give respect to the little beetle walking along, give respect to the animals, give respect to the polar bear. You give respect to all that exists by virtue of that which it is.

The essence of the thing is that which it is. And what does a thing mean? What a thing means is what it is. What it is, is what it means. That's hard to see. But then you get the essence of it. What this thing means is what it is. You don't have to add adjectives, adverbs, languaging; it speaks for itself by virtue of its existence. So, a teacher should speak for himself because of the reality of that which it is. That which it is, not that which is spoken about. It's not materialistic, not the neediness of worldly wealth and all the stuff that goes with it.

Inspirational truth avoids glamorization, seduction, and theatrics. I've been to so-called spiritual events that were like a Broadway production: videos and orchestras and flashing lights. There's no need for worldly wealth, you see. Wealth is the difference between your desires and that which you have. If you want to transcend spiritually, let go of wantingness. Let go of wanting admiration, wanting possessions, wanting control. When you finally let go of all wantingness, you've got more than what you need.

When I first came to Sedona, I rented a place. I didn't even have a bed, so I went and bought a cot at the dollar store. I bought some blankets at the Goodwill. I got a nice wooden box and put a candlestick next to it. I put an apple in the refrigerator and saved that for dinner. What more do you need? I was complete. God will provide for you if you need it, so I tested that out too. I walked out with no money or no food and wandered around Sedona. I got invited for breakfast. I got invited for lunch and invited for dinner. I'd say, "I haven't got any money." And they'd tell me it's on the house. What you need is provided. Therefore, if you need nothing, you already have abundance.

INTEGRITY OF THE TEACHER

The integrity of the teacher speaks for itself. Some people can intuit it, and other people, of course, cannot. With everything I say, I am constantly aware all the time, in an unspoken constant awareness, that I'm responsible and answerable to almighty God for everything that I say every second. And as a teacher, that responsibility is heightened. I'm extremely aware of everything I say. Therefore, very often, like when I give a lecture, I will sort of intuit a thing as being so, but I want to make sure it's so. I'll do muscle testing and say, "Let's check this out and see if it's so, because I do not want to teach any error."

I still get wild, crazy e-mails. Every author gets crazy mail, you know, where they accuse you of being a fraud in some way. And I'll say, "Having taught the whole world how to discern truth from falsehood in a matter of seconds, I'm very unlikely to try to present falsehood." Having already told them how to discern the difference between truth and falsehood, I'm not very likely going to present falsehood with tens of thousands of people out there doing that. So spiritual reality is educational, it's self-supporting. We don't ask anything of anybody except the cost of the event.

God is void of induced unnatural states of consciousness, such as parapsychological states, or the abnormal breathing patterns, positions, postures, and other ways to try and force the Kundalini energy. When the Kundalini is ready to rise, it does so automatically because of its own truth.

As you become loving, the Kundalini energy rises; it's not going to rise because you cross your legs and sit in front of a picture of the Buddha and burn incense and do all kinds of mystical incantation stuff. Just try to be kindly and loving and step over the beetle, and you can save yourself all that stuff. You can save all kinds of money on incense and mystical music and gongs. You start to see the theatricalization of it all. You get these spiritual magazines and on the cover, there's always a beautiful blonde with flowing hair. Are we supposed to believe that sexual allure is a pathway to God? After all, you never get an unattractive person on the front cover of these magazines. I thought for a while, you weren't going to get to heaven without long blond hair. They always do a mystical yoga posture too. That's the glamorization of it, the theatrics. Avoid unnatural things and especially trainings that are going to teach you mystical powers; trainings that teach you mystical powers, all of them calibrate about 205.

Look at this seduction to the spiritual ego. "Oh, I'm going to be special. And I'm going to have superpowers." If they had superpowers, they wouldn't be selling them to you, would they? If you've got superpowers, and are so rich and powerful and complete within yourself, what would you be selling it for? You'd be selling it because you're *needy*. Needy of what? More power and wealth? Give me break. I would receive so many e-mails about some weird guru somewhere, Tasmania or someplace. And the guru would calibrate at about 180.

INNER CALLING AND INNER GENUINENESS

When one is growing and seeking, there may be others in one's life that may not understand their pursuit to grow even further spiritually. Dr. Hawkins tells us how to respond in these kinds of situations.

I believe people should use discretion. You don't have to tell people what you're doing and why you're doing it. When I left the East, I didn't explain it to anybody; there's nothing they're going to understand about that. There are probably very few people who you're going to be able to confide in about what you're really up to and what's really going on with your life. Everybody has a certain comprehension of an inner calling, and I find the best way you can describe it, is "I reached a satisfaction with a certain point in my life and a very strong inner calling said to me, 'Here's a whole different other area you need develop and grow.' And I had to follow that calling."

You can usually get by with saying you have an inner calling. Of course, people will try to argue with you, because you're challenging their world view. You're negating to some degree the value of their world view. And so they may expect you to defend it. And I would not defend that. I would just say, "Look, that's my calling. And that's the way it is." "Well, what about the wife and the kids? What about the business . . ." and blah, blah, blah. I respond, "Well, God will have to look after that. God is the creator of the universe. He's the savior of mankind. God can just worry about it, because I'm going to be busy doing something else." "He's lost his mind," they'll say. Well, when your mind goes silent, you *have* lost your mind.

And I realized it's a compliment. I've been at it for 30 years; I finally did lose my mind. And they're saying, "I think he's lost his mind." Look at the life I had before. I had the life and I can't tell you how ultimate it was. It was ultimate in ways that the world doesn't even know about. The most ultimate people don't even reveal to the world what they really are about a good deal of the time. Organizations they belong to don't even appear on the map. So you walk away from that world and you walk into a different world where genuineness, intrinsic inner genuineness, is what counts. When you say thank you to a waitress or to a clerk in the store, it has to be from a genuine appreciation. You see their beingness and there is-ness. And what you're saying is the truth.

If you're just doing it as a superficial manipulation, it doesn't have the same effect. When you see how hurried the person is and how hard they're trying to keep up with it all, you appreciate the humanness in people. When you reflect back the genuine value of their humanness, what you're really reflecting back is the sacredness of their existence. You see, when you acknowledge people, you are reflecting back to them their inner worth—and their inner worth is infinite. The inner worth of every human being is infinite. Its potential is infinite.

That which is created by God . . . You can't say that one creation of God is better than another. All are equally creatures of God. So, this is the transformation you go through. Let's say you walk down the street, and you see a little black beetle on his back, flailing his legs around, and you see others walk past it. You can tell you're making spiritual progress when it bothers you, you turn the little beetle on his feet, and then you walk away happy. At that point, you realize you're loving life and you're discerning the sacredness of it, because his little life is just as sacred to him. And so you're sent by God to turn him over and say, "Well, God, I'm turning over this little beetle because I know you want me to." (You know, you can joke around with God; I do that all the time.)

There is a point where you can't walk by the beetle without helping it. Then there is an even higher space, a different level of consciousness, in which the beetle's karma is the beetle's karma, and yours is yours. So you become a servant of God when you see the intrinsic holiness of all of life and you try to preserve it as best you can, because that's how God reflects through you.

Chapter 5

SURRENDER

In this chapter, we move beyond specific spiritual obstacles to perhaps the greatest challenge that faces any spiritual seeker: the willingness to surrender everything, including the payoffs to the ego, to God.

This sounds like it would be easy. After all, to surrender means to let go and not have to do anything. What could be easier? In truth, the process of surrendering is one of the most difficult steps along the path to enlightenment because the tentacles of the ego, even among the most spiritually inclined, are deep and firmly entrenched. However, after reading this chapter, you'll see why a commitment to this surrendering process is more than commensurate with the demands.

The willingness to surrender the payoff of the ego allows you to let everything go experientially as it arises. This includes the payoff of grief, anger, resentment, or hatred. With surrender, you have to choose. What do you surrender to God in the way of surrender? What does devotion mean? I love thee, oh Lord, greater than. I love the glee I get out of my hatreds, my wickedness, my shame, my guilt, my revenge. Either you love God or you love revenge. You can't have them both. Either you love God or you love self-pity. It's always really a choice. Am I willing to surrender this for the love of God, or not? To become enlightened, that power has to be strong. You have to be willing to give up *everything* for God. And I mean everything. This is because at the last moment before that ultimate experience reveals itself (or condition takes over, rather), you will be asked to surrender your life.

The core of what you think is your life—the core of the ego, the self, the *real* you—you lay that down for God. It's scary because you need to let go of all this payoff, and you look at all this stuff. Now suddenly, there's an infinite presence that is like yourself, what you think is yourself. And this one, too, lies down, and there's a moment of terror and you experience death. There's only one death. You never experience it again. But there is one death you'll live through. You don't know that you're going to live through it.

The ego has the notion that it's going to be the same, only enlightened. "I'll still be me, but I'll be the *enlightened* me." No, you aren't going to be you. It's my responsibility to prepare you for the last moment, because everybody here is going to be headed for the last moment. Unless you hear the truth, you won't know what to do. Therefore, karmically I am laying down that I have spoken the truth. At that last moment you will get, "Walk straight ahead no matter what." Die for God. And as you lay down your life, the agony of death arises (and it is agonizing and you do die). And then, before you stands the splendor. That what you thought was life was not life anyway. But because it is so real, you see why you've guarded it all these lifetimes. It's so convincingly real, *that it is your life.* That it is the *source* to your life. The ego is very, very strong or it wouldn't have survived all these lifetimes. At this last moment, it tells you, or you feel that it's the very source of your life that you're laying down. At that point, I'm telling you, it is safe to surrender. It is safe, but you have to have a knowingness that it's safe. You have to have heard it, you have to know it. You have to have it in your aura. And then out of nowhere, it comes to you, and you walk right through. The Zen saying to walk into fear no matter what got me through it. "No matter what" means without limitation, even to death itself, no matter what. I repeat the words of the master, who I followed at that moment: *no matter what.*

• • •

As you surrender, as you're willing to let go, you'll see the ego hangs on because it's getting something out of it. Now, everybody's ego is going to resist this. Expect it to. The old ego says, "This hatred is justified." To give up self-pity, to give up anger, to give up resentment, to surrender them through forgiveness. The power of *A Course in Miracles* is the willingness to forgive all and get out of the lower fields of consciousness.

In the beginning, the ego identifies with form. How does the ego know that? Because it registers form through recognition. You'll notice that there isn't any *me* that's thinking anyway. There is a watcher-experiencer. In meditation or in contemplation, if you focus on the field, you'll notice that witnessing is happening of its own accord.

The first thing you notice about consciousness is it's automatic. The light of consciousness is automatic. It expresses as the watcher or the experiencer through awareness, the observer; you get to the source of that faculty, and you'll see that's an impersonal faculty. There isn't any personal you that decided to be consciously aware. Witnessing is happening of its own accord. In meditation you pull back from identifying with the content of meditation. *I am this, I did that*, and all that. That's all fallacious story. You realize that, that which I am is the witness of all those thoughts, feelings, and that panorama. I call it a phantasmagoria.

My great-aunt used to have something that was really special for my birthday. She called it a monster polypheme. I said, "What's that under there?" She said, "That's a monster polypheme." It would be something like a whole croquet set or something: a monster polypheme. This whole phantasmagoria that goes through the mind, everybody who has meditated knows that. Memories, thoughts, fantasies, imaginations. You realize that what you are is the involuntary witness. You don't volunteer to be the witness; you *are* the witness. No point to take credit for it, no point to feel ashamed about it because it's automatic. Consciousness automatically is conscious because that's its nature, and it's impersonal. That's part of your karmic inheritance, to be conscious.

One begins to identify with the witness, the observer, then with consciousness. Then one stops identifying that consciousness is personal, and one even goes beyond the manifest and realizes the ultimate is beyond all form, beyond manifest . . . out of which consciousness arises and that makes you a buddha.

• • •

The willingness to surrender positionality out of humility to God means that one is then ready to accept the possibility that intrinsically, men are innocent and that they're suffering from a profound ignorance and that the only way out of suffering, then, is to transcend that ignorance to your spiritual truth. Then one becomes a student of spiritual truth in their personal life, or even eventually in their professional life. The relief for human suffering then is what medicine is about, psychiatry is about—it's why I went into psychoanalysis. Each of those things was to sharpen the capacity to assist in the relief of human suffering and all of its forms, whether it's psychopharmacology or understanding unconscious conflicts. If you're dedicated to that endeavor, one eventually ends up with spiritual truth and spiritual programs, because to many human dilemmas, there is no other answer. Just like there's no other answer to the death of a loved one, except to surrender to God and the will of God in the knowingness that eventually spiritual truth will heal all pain. The way we transcend all of that again goes back to humility, and the willingness to let go of the way we see things, and allow a spiritual truth which comes in of its own. People don't realize that when one becomes silent, out of that silence, all of a sudden arises a realization.

We try to force an answer, or force God to give us an answer with a demand. Many prayers are nothing but demands. We try to force God to respond to our demand, which is disguised as a prayer. "I prayed to such and such." No, you were trying to force God to give you a new Ford. When we actually surrender to God's will, suddenly, we see it differently. And when we see it differently, we realize there is no loss. The source of the pain disappears. And when the source of the pain disappears, the source came out of ignorance and came out of the way you were seeing it. By constant surrender to God, all things resolve themselves—even very advanced and complicated, spiritually difficult issues. The best way to handle a prayer for a Ford is to surrender your desire for a Ford. Why did you want the Ford? Because you think that happiness is something outside of yourself. *If I have the new Ford, then I will feel successful and then I will feel happy.* All desires then have associated with them the unconscious belief system that they will bring us happiness, but that makes us very dependent on the external world. And so, our happiness is always vulnerable and we live in fear all the time, because if the source of happiness is outside yourself, you're always in a weakened, possibly victim, position.

If the source of happiness is self-fulfillment *within* oneself, then nobody can take it away from you. You reach a point when whether you physically live or die is really irrelevant. Many times you're looking death in the face, and if you leave, you leave, and if you don't, you don't, and it's no big deal. When we get beset by a desire, we've set ourselves up for suffering. And therefore, if we're willing to surrender everything to God, we're willing to surrender everything and anything no matter what, even life itself. Then, it's resolved and something replaces it, but it's better than the new Ford would have been.

• • •

It's the future that's creating your present. You think it's your past that's propelling you from the past, that you're being pushed by your past. No, you're being sucked into your future. You're being pulled by destiny because by an act of the will, you've already chosen your destiny, and now this is the unfolding of what is required to reach it. Therefore, there's no point to complain about it, unless you want to. (Do not feel guilty about complaining.)

How does one transcend the ego? First of all, there is no such thing as the ego. There's only the tendency of these energies to form a structure. There's only a *tendency.* They can be easily undone. There's two ways: meditation and contemplation, with prayer and devotion. Be one with the field. If you are aware primarily of the field, see if your obsessive compulsive side gets so caught up in this thing here, that it drives you crazy. He's got to know every little detail, which is totally irrelevant. Was your lunch $1.32 or $1.37? I don't know—who cares?

The I, the sense of the self: this is the vision of the totality. You live in the infinite space in which everything is happening. To be focused on, you might say, peripheral vision rather than central vision is to be aware of the totality of the situation. The entirety of all that's being here, and the energy of us being here, and what that means for what should be said here, and what should be heard for, speaks of its own. It's about the totality of the energy and the totality of beings here and their collective drive.

If you move around in the peripheral world, you're always focused on the totality of the situation, and unfortunately, you miss a lot of the details. It's best to be married if you do this. Who tells you that you put the shirt on with the hole in the sleeve? *Oh geez.* I thought, *She'll never see that. It's my favorite shirt.* In my spouse's world, you cannot wear a shirt if it has a hole in it. In my world, nobody notices it. Why? Because I pay attention to the field all the time. You can do the same thing in meditation, where you're constantly aware of consciousness itself. The opposite way is to focus on the content. There is another form of meditation or contemplation in which there is an absolute fixity of focus on the immediate present as it arises with no selection. Intensely focused on the head of a pin constantly. You're staying intensely focused in the intense now. Peripheral and central vision, the retina is sort of set up that way too, with your focus on the macula or the field.

Devotional non-duality means that the love for God is enough that you're willing to surrender everything that stands in the way of the realization of the presence of divinity, which turns out not to be an *other*, but the Self. You thought it was going to be out there later. It's a source of one's existence to come to the realization, the radical reality of subjectivity. We take subjectivity for granted. We take the field for granted. We take consciousness for granted. This is what we take for granted. This is what we think is important. This is what's trivial and irrelevant, and this is what you are. We ignore what we are in return for focusing on that which we are not.

At this very instant, 99 percent of your mind is silent. The reason you don't notice it is because you're focused on the 1 percent that's noisy. It's like you have a vast amphitheater that seats 400,000 people. Nobody's there in the middle of the night, but over in the corner, there's one little tiny transistor radio. That's what you're focused on. The whole amphitheater is empty, there's nobody in the seats, but you think *this* is where the action is. You're focused on the tiny thing of the moment attracting your attention. Because your attention is focused here, you think that's what your mind is. That's not what your mind is. The mind is the absolute silence. If your mind wasn't silent, you wouldn't know what you were thinking about. If it wasn't for the silence in the woods, you couldn't hear any noise.

How could you hear a bird sing? It's only against the background of silence. It's only against the background of the innate silence of the mind that you can witness what the mind is thinking about. At that realization you call it *it* instead of *me*. It's not what my mind is thinking about, it's what *it's* thinking about. That same realization comes about with the body. When you leave your identification with the body, you see it doing what it's doing. You have nothing to do with it. Never did you have anything to do with it. It belongs to nature and is karmically propelled. It just does what it's going to do. It's as entertaining to you as anybody else; it's just a novelty.

What are the fields of realization? As things arise, then, there's a willingness to surrender them to God. There's a willingness to surrender everything as it arises. When you hear a musical note, the note rises and then it falls. As you hear the note, it has already crested and it is already falling. Surrender, then, is the willingness to let go all positionalities of everything—that it arises as it arises. Not to label it anything, not to call it anything, not to take a position about it. The willingness to surrender everything as it arises. This allows you to go through major surgery without anesthesia. The minute you call it pain, the minute you say, "You're cutting my thumb off," the minute you start to *resist* the pain, the pain is excruciating. The minute you get off your position, but you stay on the edge of the knife, and let go of resisting, you can disappear any illness as it arises. If you fall down and you feel you've just twisted your ankle, you can't call it pain, you can't call it a twisted ankle. Let go of resisting the sensations that come up. Don't label them anything.

You're not experiencing pain; nobody experiences pain. Pain is a label. You can't experience diabetes, you can't experience pneumonia, you can't experience any of those things. Those are words, labels. You can cough, you can't *experience* a cough. That's another word you put on it. There's a sensation. You let go resisting the sensation. Completely surrender it to God, the willingness to surrender everything to God as it arises. As it arises, the willingness to surrender, it brings you into a state of Alwaysness, of the presence of reality as the source of existence.

• • •

The ego tends to think in terms of cause and effect. It thinks of goals, of achievement, of going there, and of becoming something greater. It never dawns on the ego that you are being attracted. It isn't that you're being propelled; it's that you intuit somehow some kind of a destiny within yourself, and you now find yourself attracted and interested. You're not being propelled by the past so much as attracted by the future.

The whole concept of *allowing* is foreign to our culture. Our culture thinks in very yang terms—try harder, push yourself harder. The awareness of the presence of God is really a consequence of a very yang type of positioning yourself. Yang is like striving and getting and trying harder, and it's very causal on its effect. Spiritual awareness occurs by a revelation.

Spiritual awareness occurs by a revelation.

It's like you stand back and spread your arms to the sides and say, "To thee, Oh Lord, do I surrender my thinkingness, my opinionness, my feelingness." And you appeal to divinity, and you then create the opening in a very yin inner psychic posture of allowing God to reveal. This is very well known, of course, in the 12-Step program, which is worldwide. Through studying meditation, we become conscious and aware of God's will for us. That's a supplication; that's an acceptance. Spiritual effort is not wasted.

When we talk about supplication, we talk about surrendering your life to God. When we speak of prayer, we speak of devotion—acts of devotion like pleading with God, asking to be led. There's a great deal of information that is accumulated over the centuries on how to facilitate the emergence of this capacity to be with the presence of God. There's also the inner pathway of knowledge. Of course, what the books I've written have to do with is sharing knowledge that would be propitious and help the person to unveil the inner state, which stands waiting. The inner state stands waiting—all you have to do is remove the blocks to the awareness.

Therefore, the information I give tries to undo the blocks just through knowledge. It's really the pathway of self-knowledge. And of course, specifically the thing that stands in our way is the ego. Consciousness research has to do with discerning that exact nature of the ego through comprehension of how it works and how it originated. You can begin to relinquish it. The first awareness we try to make is to realize that there's a difference between perception and essence. Of course, Descartes pointed that out centuries ago. There is the world the way you see it, and therefore, how you perceive it and how you think about it is your opinion. And then there's the world the way it actually is, which is independent of what you think about it or how you label it or what your opinion is.

The spiritual work is to try to transcend perception and begin to experience the essence of things. I think the calibrated scale of consciousness speeds that up tremendously once you've learned how to use it. Even if you look at a few lists of the calibrated levels of various things in our world, you begin to intuit it. You go, "Aha!" Underneath the sheep's clothing is what's *really* there. Inside the Trojan horse you begin to stop falling for the facile and foolish. And of course, we live in a media society in which perception eclipses everything—how a person looks on stage, et cetera. People are very impressed by that rather than by the quality and the substance of the speaker.

• • •

When a major catastrophe comes about, I'm concerned with the psychological and emotional suffering of people who are in that situation, and I pray for the relief of their anxiety and fear, because even if the crisis is always the same, depending on the circumstances, people think that it's different. Actually, an acute crisis is always the same no matter what the occasion is. Shock and surprise, disbelief, and in the middle of it, you really don't think, you don't really get upset about it until it's over. A crisis is so fast in its onset, unexpected, it's over before you know it. Then very often comes the fear—it's surprising the fear doesn't come up until the whole event is over. And then there's a quick rerun and the fear comes up at the rerun; at the time of the accident, there wasn't any fear. You handle the energy of the emotion. You handle the energy and not the quality, the energy of it.

All you have to do is surrender to the emotion, to the energy itself, and let go of resisting the energy—the energy will take care of itself. Don't forget that you have also the wisdom of the collective unconscious. If you don't remember how to handle something, the collective does, because mankind has lived through an innumerable number of crises. And in the collective awareness and consciousness of mankind are all the tools you'll need. You surrender into your humanness, and we often do that when we pray for God. That's all we do—we just suddenly come into the wisdom, accept the wisdom of the collective consciousness of all of mankind, which, of course, over the millennia has learned how to handle every crisis that's imaginable.

Don't resist the emotion and instead say, "Of course you're going to be upset. Of course you're going to be worried. Of course you're going to say to yourself, 'Oh, what are we going to do now?' Of course, you're going to go into a panic." Let it be okay to have those emotions. Those are just natural responses. They're just part of humanness. You don't have to label it that *you* are responding that way. It's *humanness* that's responding that way. The average human will go through a period of dismay, panic, fear, and then, of course, they will start making plans and discussing in their own mind what reparative steps they're going to take to ensure survival now that they've, say, lost their job.

Otherwise, what happens is one of these phases becomes protracted. You get stuck in grieving, or you get stuck in fear, or you get stuck in resentment. That's not due to worry, fear, or anger. The problem there is one of stuckness: why are you unwilling to move on?

I would point out to a patient, "Well, what are you getting out of this constant resentment?"

The patient would say their wife has left them or their boss has fired them or something, but they're milking it. I wanted them to see that they're milking it. I would tell them, "Well, that was a couple of years ago. It's time to get over it." That they're milking it, feeding off of it, and they're using it. They begin to see that they are indeed propagating the resentment themselves.

In our present society, the competition is for victimhood. It's almost hilarious how people want to rush onstage to tell you how they're the victim. And they're almost in competition to see who's the most wronged. Who's the most wronged gender or race or color? Who's a victim of money, social position, politics? Everybody's out there in the competition to see who has been the most wronged.

It's like a moral competition. Who's the most wronged here? Is it the old people or the young people? The Republicans or the

Democrats? Who's getting the biggest part of the wrong? It's almost comical when you see it. Everybody just loves to rush on television and say how they've been wronged. That's narcissism—to milk everything for all you can get out of it. And then when you finally see it for what it's worth, and you see it through the viewpoint of the self-feeding of narcissism, you only feel sorry that people got stuck in it. It's one thing to, as a passing phase, milk a crisis for all it's worth, but then there's a time to get over it. What you want to do is help people get over it and move on in life.

MOVING TO THE CONSCIOUSNESS LEVEL OF HOPE

Dr. Hawkins says that problems are not handled on the level at which they seem to be occurring, but on the next higher consciousness level. Here, he'll tell us why.

Grief can't be handled on the level of grief. You look at the levels of consciousness and you see where you're at, and then you move up. From grief or resentment or something like that, you can move up to acceptance and stop personalizing it. It's not you; it's the nature of life. It's the nature of protoplasmic life. It's the nature of human life. It's the nature of life in this country at this time. The employment rate has nothing to do with you personally. These are all personal phenomena. You learn to sort of generalize it, and not take it personally and move up to the next level of consciousness, which is hope.

When you lose one job, instead of dismay, anger, resentment, and depression, you move up to neutral. You move into thinking, *So I lost this job—so what?* You look at job listings, and there are lots of jobs. You walk down the street, and there are a lot of jobs. The town I live in, you can walk down any street in the business district and you'll see help wanted signs. Right in the middle of the great unemployment crisis, there's help wanted signs in practically half the stores. Everybody wants help. People don't want to work those hours, or for that kind of money, or under those conditions. But if you let all that go, you'd be happy to walk down the street and make good money every single day washing windows. You just see that it's not really a financial problem, but it's one of choice that you really don't want to move to the level of window washer. You want to do what you want to do—play piano, dance, paint beautiful pictures—and still get rich. Instead, you can move up to hope that this is the opening for a new, exciting adventure. You don't know what the adventure is going to be, and you don't know what kind of a job you're going to come up with.

I find every job has things that are interesting about it. No matter what kind of a job you have or where, there are always new people to meet. One of the exciting things about any new job is meeting all these new people with whom you're going to be working and getting acquainted with them. There's new friendships to be made, new associations to be made, new people who are interesting or entertaining. Some people you meet are going to be funny, and some people are going to be awful. You know that, and it's just a new adventure. Life goes from one adventure to another adventure. It's always a new adventure, living one day at a time.

THE POWER OF THE MIND IN CRISIS

A woman received a letter that her son was missing in action and she went into a depression. She stopped talking, she stopped eating, and she just rocked back and forth in her rocker. Nothing you did or said could persuade her. She wouldn't eat; she wouldn't talk. A week later, there was another letter from the war department that there had been an error. It wasn't her son who had been killed. It was somebody with the same name, with just one letter off. Her son was Phillip with two L's, and the other guy was Philip with one L. Due to a misspelling, she was misinformed. After being told that her son had not died, she showed no visible reaction at all. Everybody said to her, "Granny, granny, he's not dead. It was all a mistake." And she went on rocking, looking off into space.

It took therapy to get her out of that state. When the state took over, you might say it released all the grief of many lifetimes, which hit her all at once. Once a state comes on strongly, it then has a life of its own. It gains dominance, and it's almost like you're possessed by another spirit. Some latent spirit in your unconscious takes over and begins to dominate the field.

You see that with people with resentments too. They're resentful and angry, and when you ask them how long ago that was, they tell you, "It was 20 years ago." Twenty years ago! It's time to get off it. You've been juicing it for 20 years. What you do is you make the person conscious of the gain that they're getting out of clinging to it, and you get them to move off of it. But people will cling to injustice; they're great about injustice. They get so much gain out of being wronged that the competition is really to see who's the most wronged.

CRISIS PRAYER

"Please be with me and show me how to surrender and handle this experience."

That's a very good prayer. Any prayer in which you are calling forth the will of God, calling upon God for help, is useful. If you calibrate the energy of the event before and after you do this prayer, you see that the prayer is uplifting: it does bring forth a great deal of healing energy, and you'll come out of something that you would not have come out of before.

It helps to live in the present. Many people are living in a fearful state of expectation, and they're getting a payoff from that. Then they find out where in life they picked up this habit of fearfulness, and see all these things reflect an unawareness of the presence and the availability of God and divine help. If you think you're all alone against the impossibilities of this world, you tend to be fearful. Once you discover that you're not alone, that the presence of God is a source of help, that fearfulness disappears because you begin depending on God instead of your ego.

What you're really seeing is that your ego in and of itself is incapable of handling this whole deal. God is the source of life, and God is the source of strength, hope, and awareness. You pray to God, you surrender to God, and you say, "Well, God, I've done all I can do about it." In the meantime, you keep digging in the garden and settling back, expecting that magically the radishes are going to suddenly sprout out of the ground. It takes *your* effort. Divine help is available at all times, but you don't discover it until you surrender to it. Then you find that the energy of God handles the thing you prayed about for you. You don't have to handle it yourself. When you let it go, you realize it gets handled without your help at all.

God didn't really need you at all. You were just a witness to what was happening. And if karmically, you're destined to leave the world at this time, you gracefully leave the world at this time. What's the point of crying about it and struggling and doing an infantile kick with your little tiny toes up in the air? If it's your time to leave, leave already. If not now, later. That does take a rather profound spiritual experience: the experiential awareness of that which you really are, the Self with a capital S, is beyond life, and that death has no beginning, has no ending, and is not made of the same dimension of that which begins and ends. It's a different dimension, and knowing that your reality is not the personal self, but some essence within you that is *beyond* the personal self, out of which the sense of a personal self arises, but independent of the personal self.

If we put you to sleep with hypnosis or anesthesia or something, would you cease to exist? No, it's just your conscious awareness of yourself as a self with a small s. Once you experience the Self with a capital S, the fear of dying disappears forever. That which you are is not subject to either birth or death. It always is, always has been, always will be, and is eternal. And that which we call divinity is the essence of God within you. The source of life is the essence of divinity within you.

Imagine if I said, "You're going to die within five minutes," and you said, "Well, what do you know? I *thought* today was going to be an interesting day." If you completely surrender to it, the fear disappears. Fear is not a necessity. Fear is an accoutrement that we add onto it. It's what the narcissistic ego adds on. What could be more awful to an egocentric, narcissistic ego than the thought that it won't exist or it isn't very important.

LETTING GO OF FEAR

There is a habit of the mind that believes that if it hangs onto the fear, it will derive something that will aid its survival—and that there's some gain to the emotionality. There is the gain to the emotionality; the best thing to do is to surrender to the emotion itself. If you do that, it'll dissipate itself. If you allow fear to just completely overwhelm you, and you surrender to the fear, within surprisingly short order, the fear disappears and it becomes a "so what?" It's an awareness you really only reach through meditation, in a way. That every emotion, no matter what it is—fear, anger, resentment, contentment, love, et cetera—arises. Then you become aware of what it is that it's arising from, what it is that it's reflecting. It's because you're trying to go through the self with a small s—the egocentric, narcissistic ego—and get to the real Self. That's a little more sophisticated. Very often it takes years of meditation to do that.

And then suddenly in one instant, that which you consider your reality functions spontaneously, autonomously without you. That which you consider the *you* is not even involved. At that point very often, you leave the body or you no longer experience yourself as the body or in a body or having a body, and you become the witness of the body. And then at that point, not only do you not value your body, it doesn't seem interesting. The first time you leave the body, you're amazed. There's the body lying there. And you think, *Gee, I'd be concerned about that.* But you aren't. It's just the dumb thing lying there. It's *a* body, but it's not my body, it's not *me*. It's not particularly interesting.

• • •

We feel fear as an emotion. Obviously, we are the ones who are creating it. However, the mind does this out of habit. You're supposed to be afraid of this, you're supposed to be afraid of that. A lot of our fears are really programmed. Sickness, old age, suffering, death, and poverty are universal human fears. The ones that are reality based are based on the temporality of human life and the vulnerability of the physical body, so they're not completely irrational. We're not talking about eliminating normal survival caution, but caution is different than fear. When you're walking down certain streets in New York City, if you don't use caution, you won't be around too long. Caution is a part of wisdom. But caution is different than fear; caution has a rationality to it. Fear can arise, as everyone who has ever had a nightmare knows, out of nowhere, with a sudden panic.

We're not talking about eliminating normal self-preservation; we're just talking about irrational fears. A lot of them you get over by facing them. I always tell people who have a fear of public speaking that I had a fear of public speaking for many years. I couldn't speak. One time I was forced into having to speak in front of an audience. I was really quite anxious. Then suddenly I said something funny, and the minute the audience started to laugh, my fear disappeared. So, I made the magic discovery, and I have spoken hundreds of times since then. That was because I discovered that humor relieves all anxiety. Putting something funny in what you're saying, if it can be accomplished, will relieve your fear. The minute the audience laughs, you feel okay. That's a magical moment, that discovery. I discovered it by accident.

If there's sufficient danger in the environment, as we said, exercising caution is a rational, survival technique. What we're talking about are fears that have no basis in reality. Overcoming them takes a certain degree of courage and a willingness to plunge into them. I think the average person doesn't have any trouble differentiating the two. With any feeling, if you stop avoiding it and plunge into it and say, "I want more of it," and let it run its course, you will eventually run it out. And sometimes you can do this with imagination. You imagine what it is you're afraid of, and you let the fear come up and you let go resisting the fear. Well, there is a limitation to the amount of any emotion. And if you keep coming up with what you're afraid of, eventually you'll run out of fear, and you'll find it's almost impossible to make yourself afraid of the next thing that you bring up to be afraid of. You can run out an emotion by letting go of resisting it—you decompress it. Then you ask yourself, *What else am I afraid of? What else am I afraid of?* until finally you run out of things that you can imagine yourself being afraid of.

One thing you can control is *focus*. For example, you can think about your toes. I might tell someone who is afraid of public speaking, "When you go up on that stage and are standing behind the podium, I want you to think about your toes while you're there." Well, if you try that, you'll find you can't be afraid because you're too busy thinking about your toes. And eventually that makes you laugh, and the minute you laugh, your fear disappears. Think about your toes. Once in a while when I want to give a lecture, there's some authors' names I always forget. I picture those names as being written on my toes. When I can't think of them during a lecture, I look down at my toes, and suddenly I remember.

I've done this many times with people who have public speaking phobias, and I have them practice at home and practice with me. Public speaking is probably the most common phobia I've gotten requests for. I take people through the whole experience—to keep imagining and letting go until finally, they run out of fears. You'll run out of fear. There's always so much fear that's compressed, but you can run it out.

AND THEN WHAT?

If you have a fear of something, use a technique I call, "And Then What?" When you do this, you keep surrendering at each level.

For example, you say, "If I lose this job, then I won't have enough money to live on."

Then you say, "And then what?"

"If I don't have enough money to live on, then I'll lose my house."

And you say, "And then what?"

"Well, if I lose my house, then I've got to rent an apartment somewhere."

"And then what?"

"And then if I don't have any money at all, I'll have to move out of the apartment too."

"And then what?"

"I won't have enough money to buy food."

"And then what?"

"And then I'll starve to death."

You think to yourself, *How are you going to do that? Are you going to sit on the sidewalk and starve to death?*

"And then what?"

"And then I'll get a tin cup and hold it up and beg for money."

"And then what?"

"And then people will laugh at me as an idiot, sitting out there with a tin cup."

"And then what?"

"And then the cops will come and take me away."

"And then what?"

"They'll decide I'm crazy."

"And then what?"

"And then they'll put me in a mental hospital."

"And then what?"

"And then I'll have a psychiatrist."

You keep doing the "And Then What?" technique, and as you surrender to the "and then what" scenarios, you disappear into absurdity and get to the bottom of the fears. *I'll be poor and ugly, and nobody will like me and nobody will hire me.* And you keep going with "and then what" until you hit the bottom of it. You'll eventually run out of "and then what" scenarios. There's a stack, so work through the stack.

I had an unexpected experience while riding in a hot air balloon across the Grand Canyon. I thought I was going to be terrified the whole time. What happened was, as I looked over the side, I just let the fear keep coming up. And I ran it out. I ran out of fear. I didn't know you could run it out. I thought that it would be a permanent thing that I would always be afraid of a certain experience, but I discovered that you can run it out. People are amazed—they think it's going to be there permanently. It won't. Keep running it, and sometimes by introducing music you can change the emotional coloration of a memory. To review that memory in the face of some kind of music that has the opposite effect; it can have quite a dramatic impact that changes the entire field.

The thing that raises it the most, of course, is turning a situation over to God. Prayer and turning a thing over to God is the strongest. I remember when I was facing a rattlesnake. There I was all alone, and I suddenly came upon this rattlesnake, and he was all coiled up and ready to go. I surrendered to God at great depth. I just let go and surrendered into the knowingness of the presence of God, and a profound peace overcame both the rattlesnake and me. It was like we were suspended in time, in a state of peaceful tranquility, sort of a Shangri-La magicalness.

The snake was calm and peaceful, and I was calm and peaceful. Both of us relinquished our fear of each other, because the snake was afraid of me too. But both of us were suspended, and there was a feeling of profound stillness, calm, peace, and timelessness. We managed to escape into a divine state, and that divine state, the power of it, also tranquilized the rattlesnake. Neither one of us moved; we were both absolutely just poised. It was a great moment. It lasted on temporal time, a matter of seconds probably. But in experiential time, it was timeless.

Invoking divinity, of course, is the most powerful way to transform it. On the other hand, you can't dictate to God how you want divinity to occur. That's what I think is traditionally called *outlining*: telling God how you want it done, when, and with whom. When you surrender, that means you surrender the outcome and say, "Whether I get this job or not, I surrender it to God." Well, then, you can't turn around and complain that you didn't get the job. It would be okay if you got it, and it'd be okay if you didn't. If you don't get the job it's because God wants you to work elsewhere. You win either way.

Chapter 6

TRUTH

The next chapter serves to answer one of life's most profound spiritual questions: What is truth? After all, in this age of the Internet we are living in, you can find many, many blogs and websites from so-called authorities or gurus claiming to speak the truth on any number of subjects. And often, these claims conflict or outright contradict one another. So again, what is truth?

In the text that follows, taken from Dr. Hawkins's Truth vs. Falsehood *program, Dr. Hawkins discusses the "38 Characteristics Inherent in Spiritual Truth." After reading about these characteristics, we hope you have a deeper understanding and insight into this profound inquiry.*

#1: Truth Is Always True

Universality means that truth has always been revealed in exactly the same way throughout all of history, over thousands of years, different parts of the globe, different cultures, different ethnic settings. The realized mystic has spoken the same truth throughout all of time. In fact, it is this characteristic that has brought up doubt in the minds of some skeptics. And the skeptic who is scientific says, "On the other hand, it still troubles me that in diverse cultures, many centuries removed from each other, the same declaration is made over and over again. There must be some universality." So truth is always true at all times, in all places, to all people. It may not be discoverable, but the eventual truth that emerges is always the same truth. The truth by its nature has to be the same, no matter what, because it's not subject to personal opinion or views.

#2: Truth Is Non-Exclusionary

Truth is all inclusive. There's no secret about it. Nobody owns it. It's open for anyone to discover who wishes to do so and wishes to go through the inner discipline to discover it for themselves. It's not limited. It's available to everyone. Just like seeing the sky is available to everyone. It's not exclusive. That means that it's all inclusive. There are no secrets, it's not limited, it's not sectarian. It means that nobody owns the truth exclusively, despite the fact that many such groups peddle that claim, that they are the sole owners of truth. Nobody has any exclusive ownership of the truth any more than they have exclusive ownership of sunlight or the sky.

#3: Truth Is Available

It's available, because like the sky, it's open to everyone. It's not exclusive. There are no secrets to be revealed, nothing to be sold, no magical formulas or mysteries. The sky has no mysteries. It stands open, honest, revealed.

#4: Spiritual Organization Has Integrity of Purpose

There's nothing to gain or lose. In other words, there is no profit if you go along with the organization and nothing to lose if you leave it. Why? Because truth is self-sufficient; it's self-fulfilling in and of itself. Like the state of what the world calls enlightenment or self-realization. It's complete and total; it needs nothing from anyone. It doesn't need people's agreement. It's complete and total unto itself. The truth has no needs.

#5: Truth Is Non-Sectarian

This is sort of a development of the first quality, of universality. Truth is not an exposition of a limitation. People want to claim exclusive ownership of truth. Here's this select little group that nobody has ever even heard of. They've got this great revelation from Master Baba on the other side. I mean, the whole thing's idiotic, and then they claim that this is the exclusive truth the whole world must abide by. So truth is non-sectarian; it's not limited to favorite groups.

#6: Truth Is Independent of Opinion

Truth is not subject to the intellect. Whether a thing makes sense intellectually, whether it makes sense within the linear world of form or not, is irrelevant. Theology tries to make spiritual truth fit within the explicable, the definable, and the logical, and to put it in an intellectual context. You can say something about truth, but what you say about it is not what it *is* because you're only *talking* about it. To really know truth, you have to *be* it.

#7: Truth Is Devoid of Positionality

As we mentioned, truth is not anti-anything. There is no opposite to truth; there's only its absence. Ignorance is just the absence of truth, and therefore, truth doesn't really have any enemies. Whether people believe it or not is their problem. It neither wins nor loses by affirmation.

#8: Truth Has No Requirements or Demands

In other words, truth, being self fulfilling and integrous, has nothing to peddle. There's no required memberships; you don't have to pay any dues; and there are no regulations, oaths, rules, or threats if you want to leave or not participate. Freedom, therefore, is intrinsic, which we'll get to later.

#9: Truth Is Non-Controlling

This differentiates it from what is peddled by cults in which the leader wants to control everybody down to the most minute details: their sex lives, how they should dress, whether they should have a beard or not, whether to have a hat. What would God care about whether you wear a hat or have a beard? Cults are characterized by not only control, but almost slavery.

#10: Truth Is Free of Force or Intimidation

The downside of cults is that there is progressive brainwashing. All kinds of adulation of leaders: "Oh, master so-and-so, Baba, Baba." All kinds of rituals, indoctrinations. These people are really programmed scientifically. And you say, "How could people seeking the truth be programmed to do the things they do?" People don't realize how powerful programming is. That's why there are professional deprogrammers out there—because once you've been programmed, you're blind and deaf. People who are caught in cults are in a desperate situation and can do dangerous things from force and intimidation.

#11: Truth Is Non-Binding

Spiritual truth is complete and total in itself. It has nothing to gain, so it doesn't have any regulations. It doesn't have any laws, no contracts. You don't have to sign anything. The wisdom says never go along with an oath or pledge. Why? Because you're binding yourself in more than this lifetime. All kinds of horrible things happen to people and if you research the karmic propensity, they took an oath in a lifetime. They took an oath, and the oath usually ends up, "Oh, I made the reverse be my fate." The minute you hear that, watch out, because you know what? Karmically, the reverse is going to be your fate because you just took an oath.

#12: Freedom Is Innate to Divinity

Karmically, we are the only ones who paddle our canoe; it moves by our choice and our options. So spiritual truth, then, would exhibit the quality of divinity itself, of freedom. Everything is voluntary. There's no adulation of people: people who serve spiritual organizations are the servants, and they do what they do, and there's no point in adulation and that kind of thing.

#13: Commonality

That means recognition is dependent on what you are. Your reality comes out of what you have become and what you are now, not as a result of some external addition, a title or a trapping or an office or some extraneous power. Recognition is a consequence of what you have actually become. We give people credence because we are believing in their integrity, not because they have some title.

That's in contrast to the cult leaders. The only power they have is their title, but their knowledge of truth, if you calibrate it, is usually less than 200.

#14: Truth Is Inspirational

Inspiration is different than glamorization. Many people are impressed because a teacher is called a great avatar and has millions of followers worldwide. And yet, when you calibrate that avatar, he or she calibrates at about 300. You need to look past the followers, the title, and the theatrics. There's so much costuming and posturing, and it's always popular to wear a robe and sandals and have long hair and a staff. That's the old Jesus symbol. I'm sure Jesus didn't even look like that.

#15: Truth Is Non-Materialistic

Spiritual truth is not interested in financial gain, wealth, pomp, et cetera. There are many cults. They're not rare. They're common, and they will fleece you financially and work you for money. It's really horrendous. Think about it like this: if you're complete and total within yourself, of what good would worldly wealth be? Well, what happens is the cult leader or the religion justifies it. They say, "If we have lots of money, then we can spread the good word and save the world." Sure, you and everybody else who's screwed religion out of its integrity has said exactly the same thing. "For the sake of the good Lord, you can sign over all your goods to us." And in the meantime, your wife can work for free in the kitchen and we'll take over your kids at a certain age and you can sign your property over to us right here—and now you've just saved your life. That's such thin rationalization. You wonder how anybody can say, "For the good of the faith, we need your wealth." Why is it always your wealth that they need?

#16: Truth Is Self-Fulfilling

It's already total and complete. It doesn't need to sell. So this is the counter to proselytization, propagation, advertising, and promotion.

A lot of these groups, they're peddling some simple spiritual technique. It's a simple technique, which you can, frankly, read about in any spiritual book. They'll take two sentences and build a whole program around that. And now they charge you $450 for a training weekend. In the meantime, they put out some very slick-looking advertising. You know, it's like investing in the gold market or something. These great big things that come in the mail. Then they have celebrities in there, actresses and famous names, who swear by how wonderful this particular technique is. For which, of course, there is a charge. And many of these are even marketing systems. Whether they're selling vacuum cleaners or a specific spiritual technique, the marketing is exactly the same. The strategy is the same and the advertising is the same. And they have a picture of the great leader. And then they have celebrities telling you how wonderful their lives are now.

I don't charge anything for my workshops. Now, there are the legitimate costs for publications, rental space, employees, et cetera. But what often happens is people get into the necessity of constantly peddling, commercializing, promoting, and prosely-tizing—and lose sight of the intention. What is the intention?

It's important to understand the difference between making a living and making a profit. Profit is a different concept. Every minister needs to make a living so that he can spend his time and energy helping his flock. An integrous minister obviously is supported by the congregation. To profit means he goes out to his congregation now and begins to exploit them.

#17: Truth Is Detached

Truth itself is detached from worldly affairs because truth doesn't have any dependency on worldly affairs. The degree of truth that is exhibited by worldly affairs is known, but there's no human involvement. In other words, you don't hear me saying I want to save the world. As Sri Ramana Maharishi said, surrender the world to God and keep up your egoistic intentions for what you perceive, because what you perceive doesn't even exist. That's only your perception. What you see as disaster is somebody else's salvation, for God's sake. So, if you want to turn this world into a Nirvana, it would lose its purpose. You would then have to create a whole other planet where evolving souls can come on—where there's a whole mixture of options, both positive and negative—so they can undo their negative karma and gain positive karma.

If you turn this into a celestial realm, there wouldn't be any reason for a celestial realm. It would *be* the celestial realm. So, if you envision that the purpose of this world is for the evolution of consciousness, then it's a perfect world. This world is perfect just the way it is. There's nothing to improve. If people didn't hit bottom, they wouldn't turn around, would they? So you're going to deprive them of the opportunity of hitting bottom?

My understanding of the intention of human life is it's the maximum opportunity for karmic gain. After all, the Buddha said, "rare it is to be born a human." It is extremely rare to be born a human. It is a karmic gift to be born a human. Why would we want to negate the gift of being born a human? Human life has its downsides—poverty, sickness, old age, death, grief, and loss—but in human life, you learn that. So, you keep coming back until you stop being attached to human life.

#18: Truth Is Benign

Truth is benign, because truth is identifiable along the whole calibrated level. Its opposite doesn't exist unless you demonize it. People who are fighting the absence of truth by personalizing it as the devil or evil or something are at war against an invisible enemy. How can you be the enemy of God? How can you be the enemy of the sky? That which prevails beyond all time-space locality and is not linear is not vulnerable to anything. How could it have an enemy? Does the sky have an enemy? Tell me, who's the enemy? Is it sunlight? No, truth has no enemies.

#19: Truth Is Unintentional

Truth does not intervene. It's not trying to promulgate or promote anything. Spiritual integrity is invitational but not promotional. We tell you how it is, how it was, and how it is now . . . those are the famous words. And if you wish to join us, you will be welcomed with open arms, but we have nothing to gain by promoting your participation or your belief of our systems. Nothing to promote or nothing to gain, because at that point, you've compromised yourself. Truth does not compromise itself or make itself conditional. It doesn't have anything to peddle or sell. It has nothing to gain. It is not interested in power over others.

#20: Truth Is Non-Dualistic

Everything comes about by virtue of potentiality becoming actuality when the propensities are there, when conditions are right. You see the emergence of potential being realized and coming into actuality, which is really the unmanifest becoming manifest. What you're really seeing is the unfolding of creation.

#21: Truth Is Tranquility and Peace

This is sort of a development from what we've said before—tranquility and peace, to have peace of mind. In other words, you cannot make your peace of mind dependent on consequences. You can lead them, but you can't make them drink, because otherwise you would have no peace of mind. What you *can* bring people is the truth. And then the effect is up to their karmic propensity because that's their purpose of being in this world—because people who are really aligned with truth and have arisen to a certain point are electrified the minute they hear it. The minute you hear it, you say, "That's it. Just got it."

Tranquility and peace means you're not trying to force others. You're not trying to control God. Everybody wants to help God. God doesn't need help any more than gravity needs help. The infinite field of consciousness itself is infinitely powerful.

#22: Truth Is Equality

In Chapter 1, we learned that if you like chocolate, you don't have to vilify vanilla, because all of life has its intrinsic value. And therefore, it's not a matter of being for this and against that; it's a matter of preference. You can prefer chocolate over vanilla, but that doesn't mean you have to be anti-vanilla. You see this play out in politics, and it is often so emotionally disturbing. People don't just say, "I prefer this candidate because . . . " and then tell you the wonderful things about the candidate. They vilify the opponent. And the villifiers, ironically, I think, tend to win votes for the other side.

#23: Truth Is Non-Temporal

Truth is not based in the physical. And the basic truth of all this is that life is not subject to death. Life cannot be destroyed; it can only change form. The minute you leave this body, you look down, and the body has nothing to do with you. In fact, you have to be sort of convinced to go back in it. There it lays in bed, and the body looks sick in a hospital bed or something like that. And here you are at peace and tranquility, about 20 feet away from the body.

#24: Truth Is Beyond Proof

Spiritual reality is nonlinear. That which is provable is linear. Therefore, you cannot prove spiritual truth. It's a complete subject of realization and needs no agreement, needs no verification. It needs nothing at all. It stands on its own. It can be corroborated, verified, testified to, but it cannot be proven. So that's why there's a diversity between science and spirituality. Science goes up to the door, but it can't go through the door, because to go through the door, you have to shift the paradigm. You go from the linear to the nonlinear, and in the nonlinear, which is a different paradigm of reality, it's the context instead of the content. So provability is within the content, but context is something different. And of course, the context of spiritual reality is infinite.

#25: Truth Is Mystical

Truth is mystical because it's beyond logical. It can't be intellectualized or mentalized. People go, "Oh, that's mystical." Mystical means in a different dimension, a different paradigm. Spiritual truth emerges on its own when the obstructions to it are removed. It isn't something that's constructed; therefore, it's not provable. When you remove the clouds from the sky, the sun shines forth— that's it. And removing the clouds does not cause the sun to shine.

#26: Truth Is Ineffable

Truth is not capable of linear definition. Psychologist William James wrote a very famous book, and he was the one who really introduced the term ineffable to describe religious and spiritual experiences. It's purely subjective. And what happens is the content diminishes and is replaced by pure context with no linearity. That is not describable. So, the problem with trying to describe spiritual reality is if you try to language it, the language is based on different premises, and then it's pure subjectivity. If you feel that you love something, appreciate something, et cetera, the best you can do is a sort of superficial explanation, but you can't really recreate the experience. You can't recreate it. It's ineffable.

#27: Truth Is Simplistic

Truth is simplistic because it's nonlinear. Linearity leads to complexity. Simplicity: the sky just is what it is. The sunlight is what it is. Nature is what it is. And you see the perfection of all that exists. And for a person who can't see the perfection, it's impossible to have them see it. At a certain level, you see the intrinsic, stunning beauty of all that exists. Of course, one function of the artist is to select something, some small part of life, and bring it to our attention. Take it out of the context in which it occurred, represent it in a different context. And now you can see its uniqueness and its stunning beauty. But until the artist pointed it out to you, you were oblivious to it. Edgar Degas showed the ballet dancers, resting their feet and massaging their ballet slippers. That was just the back of the theater, kind of a nothing event. When he brought that moment forth, then we saw the incredible design, and of course, he created some of the most famous paintings in the world.

#28: Truth Is Affirmative

It's beyond provability. Therefore, it's beyond opinion, and it can only be confirmed by being it. You can only *be* that. You can't confirm it or prove it. You can only know what it is to be a cat by being a cat. So you can read all the encyclopedias you want about cat-ness. When you ask the cat, "Is that describing you?" the cat says, "It's got nothing to do with who I am." You say to the cat, "Well, who are you?" and the cat says, "Me." Subjectively, we all just identify with our own existence.

#29: Truth Is Non-Operative

This is a little difficult to understand. Because it's nonlinear there's no this nor that. It's non-dualistic. Truth stands on its own. It doesn't *do* anything. You might say it's the stage, you know, like the sky doesn't do anything, it just *is*. So, the ultimate reality, which is the subject of realization, is everything's meaning is what it is. The meaning of this table is completely explained by what it is. And any mentalization about it is unnecessary. Everything means what it is. What it is, is what it means. When you say, "Who are you?" and then you say, "I'm me," that's because, you see, that is a complete and total statement. It needs no amplification.

#30: Truth Is Invitational

Spiritual truth attracts because of the power of its integrity. Cults that use coercion and intimidation and such are using *force*. Spiritual truth comes from power. And it attracts; it has a magnetic attraction to people who calibrate over 200. To people who are under 200, it may have the opposite effect, and they avoid truth because it's a different domain in which they can't survive. If your survival is based on falsehood, the last thing you want is to face ultimate truth.

#31: Truth Is Non-Predictive

Just on the physical level, we saw from the Heisenberg principle that the state of the universe, as it is now, which we can define by the Schrödinger equation, is changed by merely observing it. Because what happens is you collapse the wave function from potentiality to actuality. You now have a new reality. In fact, you have to use different mathematical formulas, like the Dirac equation. So, you've gone from potential into actuality. That transformation does not occur without interjection of consciousness. Consequently, a thing could stand as a potentiality for thousands of years. Along comes somebody who looks at it differently, and bang, it becomes an actuality. So the unmanifest then becomes the manifest as the consequence of creation. Therefore, predicting the future is impossible because you would have to know the mind of God, because creation is the unfolding of potentiality, depending on local conditions and intention. You have no idea what intention is. Intention can change one second from now. If the future was predictable, there would be no point to human existence because there would be no karmic benefit, no gain or capacity to undo that which is negative. It would be confined to what is called predestination. Predestination and predictions of the future miss the whole purpose of existence and jump the whole understanding of the evolution of consciousness. There would be no karmic merit nor demerit. There would be no salvation. There would be no heavens. There would be no stratifications of levels of consciousness. We would all just emerge perfectly in a perfect realm. And therefore, there would be no purpose to this life at all.

It's an absurdity—all of these predictions about the future are absurdities. And if you calibrate them, they're all way below 200. "Beings from the future who don't even exist yet are going to enter your realm and tell you all this and that." And, you know, it's all poppycock.

#32: Truth Is Non-Sentimental

A lot of people confuse spirituality with sentimentalism. "Oh, if we're nice to them, they're going to be nice to us," they say. I'll tell you, if you're nice to them, they're going to behead you slowly. They are not going to be nice to you. Why? Because to them, you're a nonbeliever. To them, you're a heretic, and as a heretic, you deserve to die. Sentimentalism gets mistaken for spiritual compassion. It is hand-wringing, weepy, wimpish behavior, peddled as spiritual. It's not spiritual at all. It's self-indulgent, narcissistic emotionalism. It's really childish, to be honest with you.

There is a difference between compassion and sentimentality. Compassion sees the essence of things. Sentimentality is hanging on to what it means to *you*. It's projecting your perception onto what's happening out there and then going into an emotional

103

spasm about it. When you witness death, you witness death. There's no point in worrying. You should be sufficiently non-attached. It's inevitable. Tomorrow is going to come. Everybody's wringing their hands, saying, "Oh, tomorrow is coming. Tomorrow is coming." It's self-indulgent. Sentimentality means emotionalizing, because the ego loves the drama of emotionalizing. The ego loves to be center stage in the Greek tragedy, cast as the hero. And so it's a way of being center stage in your inner make-believe theater of what your life is and what it means. The spiritual reality doesn't get any payoff from egoistic positions.

Sentimentalism is melodrama. It belongs on the stage. It's making a theater out of life.

I tell people this to prevent the pain of going in a direction that is going to bring them further pain. I know people who are still grieving the loss of a family member from 40, 50 years ago. Why? Because the payoff is so big. They want sympathy, but they're pulling energy out of everybody around them. People at that level are pulling energy out of your solar plexus. Anything under 200 is pulling your energy, and that which is over 200 is adding to your energy.

Sentimentalism is being an energy vampire. I had a person who worked at my clinic, and once she got off the phone with a client and told me, "She wants to rip out my guts with her story." I thought that was the best description of it.

Compassion has a completely different attitude. You can have sympathy for that which suffers, but you find you give that up after a while. Later, you have empathy for it. *Yes, I know how you actually feel.* And then you end up with compassion, where you don't try to influence what the other person is going through. It's theirs to suffer out, learn from, and complete the karmic lesson in it.

You can have compassion, but you don't take it on yourself. That's it. Because if you take on the responsibility, you've just joined the karmic obligation of it and the karmic consequences of it. Think about the crowds of people in the 1700s who used to watch beheadings at the guillotine. "Oh, it's only the person up there, the hangman that's getting bad karma out of doing this," we might say. No, the spectators are assuming karmic obligation. So with sympathetic participation, large numbers of people are wiped out periodically by tsunamis or floods or volcanoes. We used to attribute that to God. "God is angry or jealous." What you're actually seeing by group participation is the consequences of group karma.

Well, I hate to break it to you, but you have an obligation now. You've participated in action. The infinite field of consciousness is, like I said, a giant electromagnetic field. So within your little iron-filing magnetic body is the code for that event. That little code pulls you into a certain maelstrom of energy and you get drowned along with the rest of the crowd.

Nothing happens by accident. Universal justice. All happens as a consequence of that which it is, that which it is. So every decision then influences that which you are. The consequences that come about are a consequence of what you are. That's why God's justice is perfect and absolute. It doesn't need man's help at all. As a consequence of that which it has become, you are where you are, and you are where you are because of the energy of that field— you're attracted to it. You don't know why you were attracted to go there when you did, because it's not within the conscious recall, but the infinite power of the universe is such that if I take a magnetic field of infinite power and you have even one hair of energy on you, you're going to get sucked right over. The field is so powerful. So if you're cheering in the crowd as the guillotine falls, you have just put a hair on your karmic inheritance, and it's not by accident that you then re-experience the same thing, but in reverse.

People are attracted by the gruesome and the spectacular. That's the emotionalism, which below 200 has a powerful influence. And the more you're above 200, the less it has an influence. Car crashes are routine. "So what?" It sounds hard-hearted. It's because you've become non-attached. When you're attached, you sentimentalize. So non-attached means it can be or not be: it's irrelevant. Detached means indifferent. You don't care if they're suffering—they're in the car, and it has turned over. Non-attached means you can stop because you don't have any fear of getting sucked in. You can call 911, make sure somebody is on their way, and hang out and then leave, but you're not sucked into it. So emotionalism means getting sucked into it now energy-wise, and, of course, karmic-wise.

#33: Truth Is Not Authoritarian

One of the reasons for the emergence of secularism, the increasing popularity of secularism, especially in Europe, was because Europe had its day with ecclesiastic authoritarianism. Everybody was slaughtered because they were Protestant or because they were not Protestant. Our culture has sort of had it with authoritarianism. And one of the main reasons is it confuses authority with authoritarianism; they're two different things. Authoritarianism is the abuse of authority. Authority is a legitimate position by virtue that you've earned it. Authoritarianism doesn't require authenticity. Anybody can adopt authoritarianism as a style. To be an authority, people usually even stop being authoritarian.

As a physician, I know what's going to cure a patient. In my authority, I say, take this, because the likelihood is about 90 percent that you're going to be better in a matter of days.

Now what they do about it is their problem. I don't need to take on the karmic responsibility for their acquiescence or their disagreements. If they disagree, I will explain everything. But it's allowing others the freedom of being who they are. See, because when you intervene, you're now pulling into your own karmic energy fields, you might say. By participation, the minute you get involved in somebody else's affair, now you're taking on some karmic responsibility.

We advise our children, and because of their love for us, we hope that that will win in the end. On the other hand, everyone has lessons to learn, and it may be more important that they learn the mistake of that pathway than please their parents.

#34: Truth Is Non-Egoistic

This is counter to all the ceremonial pomp of religion, the accoutrements and the vestments and all the whole thing. I think a teacher should be respected. Students will ask, "What do you want from us?" Just respect for the truth of what I'm saying and the energy and commitment to it, to try and drive it and express it in the best way possible. That's all. The only thing I want is the same that any other integrous endeavor would bring forth. If you're a carpenter and make a good piece of furniture that will last a couple hundred years, it's good carpentry. So, all we want is acknowledgment.

That's just a matter of respect, but adulation is a play. It's really a play by the adulator. The adulator is trying to play off that which it adulates, thinking it's going to have some gain. Plus, what they're adulating is the image and the magic associated with that image and all the pomp and the ceremony. This avatar had millions of followers worldwide, and if you calibrate him, he would hardly break level 200. But he knows how to put on a show.

#35: Truth Is Educational

You try to provide the means by which any interested person can arrive at the truth on their own. You try to describe it, verbalize it, have it recorded, printed, whatever. You try to make the information available. If you discover $E=mc^2$, you want the whole world to know what the mathematics are, what the physics are, what the subparticle physics world is like, how it's designed, how it thinks. Because that's how the world grows—by each person learning about that. That's the purpose of the encyclopedia. For learning and growing. We contribute to that.

All the teacher does is contribute to the knowledge of the world and try to provide inspiration and the integrity of witnessing. So, the state itself, which replaces what was the mind, is not an occasion for grandiosity. On the other hand, neither can it be ignored. So, you give testimony to the fact that when the clouds are removed, the sun shines forth. And also that when winter hits you, you may not be able to function for quite a while at the time. So the integrous, spiritual student, should be prepared in advance for the state of immobilization. When you sit at 600 and bliss, frankly, you're going to sit on the rock and you might just fall over there. Because it's irrelevant whether the body sits there or doesn't sit there.

The reason we discussed also the pitfalls, the seduction of the innocent into a non-integrous cult and things like that, is because I think a teacher should also forewarn students of the downside. "If you're going to visit a dangerous area, hold your purse tightly to your body and don't lend it to a stranger to borrow your lipstick." It's a lot like being a parent. You forewarn them of the traps that come up, because each level of consciousness has its trap on the downside.

#36: Truth Is Self-Supporting

Truth is neither mercenary nor materialistic. Self-supporting means it charges for whatever the expenses are. If you're going to put on a conference, it is going to cost you money, and you divide it up and try to figure out what's going to make it work and whether there's a surplus left over to pay the office staff until the next one. So, it's self-propagating, and you don't have to solicit funds or do fundraising. You don't have to work people over. I hear all the time how people have been worked for the good of the cause and this and that. And they've really been worked over and exploited by salesmanship.

#37: Truth Is Freestanding

Truth's credibility does not depend on any external. Why is that? Because its authority comes from the reality of that which it is, which is purely subjective and experiential. So you don't have to quote authorities. For instance, in the books that I've written, I practically never quote an authority. You read any books on spirituality and they're just endless quotes of some other author elsewhere in time and place. Well, why don't they speak for themselves? You can mention that Socrates agrees with the same thing to give a little historical context, but quoting Socrates is not to give it authenticity, but for clarification. So you see a trend going throughout human history. The truth at that level was already available in 400 BC and hasn't really changed, and that its applicability to current spiritual life is as timely as it was then. So don't depend on making a statement by quoting an outside authority. The only reason $E=mc^2$ is because Professor Schmooglemaurer said so, and Clockenburger, you know, in 1922. It's based on his own understanding and realization. It's self-standing, so it stands on its own. So I've tried to make this work stand on its own and be reaffirmable by anybody who wishes to track it.

#38: Truth Is Natural

Because of that which you have become, the Kundalini energy flows automatically based on the level of consciousness through the appropriate chakra system, the acupuncture system, and it alters the brain physiology as a consequence of that which it is. Remember that from 200 and up, brain physiology shifts the left brain to the right brain. And the whole sequence of processing is completely different. This is natural. It's a consequence of that which you have become. If you turn your life into devotion to become that, and you *be* that, as a matter of being that, then when you can see the beauty and divinity of all that exists and the sacredness of all of life, et cetera, and you see the divinity that shines forth through all of creation, you try to imitate it. So altered. You see a lot of these strange energy manipulation systems. I saw one on television the other night; it was supposed to be levitation or something like that. I mean, it was ridiculous. If you calibrate, it's got nothing to do with levitation. Levitation, having gone through the siddhis myself, I can tell you, it has nothing to do with what you do whatsoever. It has nothing to do with how you breathe, or whether you picture lights flowing around you, recite peculiar things, or breathe through one nostril or the other. The siddhis, which can happen at a certain level of consciousness, flow up your back, like an exquisite energy. This energy sponta-neously in and of that which it is flows into the world. And all the so-called paranormal phenomena happen automatically as a con-sequence of their own. It has nothing to do with you personally. To try and force these things unnaturally can be catastrophic.

And you may have read about Kundalini psychosis, or the stu-dents whose energy went up one side and not the other and they were lopsided and staggered over and were sick for years, et cet-era. And this is trying to force the Kundalini energy. The spiritual energy is divine energy. What you're trying to do is force God's hand: "I'll just breathe this energy up into this chakra and then I'll be such and such." Why don't you just be such and such and then the energy will fill up to that chakra? It's like trying to drive the horse with the buggy. No, that which you've become automat-ically pulls to itself that which is concordant with that, which it is. To try and force it unnaturally, I don't advise.

You can go the whole gamut, the evolution of consciousness, and along the way, there are no others, no angels that speak to you or archangels. No visions, no voices coming out of trees. No whis-perings from the grass, no monkeys suddenly beginning to talk.

There's no master on the other side. There's no other entity, even at the very highest level where you have to surrender your life itself—there's no *other* there. When you have to make the most major decision possible, in the evolution of consciousness, there's no other to guide you. No other, no guardian angel, no Baba. There's nobody there. You're absolutely all by yourself. The only thing that accompanies you is a frequency and an energy in the aura. That's the grace of the guru, the traditional grace of the master. So, the high spiritual teaching shines forth as a frequency vibration, a very high frequency vibration in your aura. That's the silent transmission, but it's not a personage. It is a frequency and an energy of the knowingness, which comes forth, not from elsewhere, but from within oneself as a knowingness, because all spiritual evolution is a revelation. All fear is an illusion. Walk through it. And that knowingness, because you're giving your life itself, comes with a very high frequency vibration. The power of it has to be greater than the power of the ego. The ego's been around a long, long time. Millennia. Long before mankind was even thought of. The ego ruled in the energy of that energy. There better be a knowingness on the most profound level. Turn over your life to the unknown and walk through a gate.

With truth, there's no reliance on externals. You can't turn your life over to an unseen entity on the other side, either calibrated or not calibrated. Most of them on the other side are into holding power over you—why would they be hanging out instead of going on into celestial realms? You don't suddenly hear a voice saying, "I'm Master Hookah. I'm 35,000 years old. Follow me." No, doesn't happen that way. Because it is tricky. On the other hand, it's so simple.

Chapter 7

THE 9 FUNDAMENTALS
OF CONSCIOUS
SPIRITUAL GROWTH

In the last few chapters, we cleared out the obstacles to spiritual growth, the tentacles of the ego, and the false ideas that some try to disguise as spiritual truths. Now, we're going to, as great educators or athletic coaches say, go back to basics. The section that follows, taken from Dr. Hawkins's audio program, In the World But Not Of It, *will outline the nine fundamentals of conscious spiritual growth. Focus on and apply these fundamentals to your life, and if you do nothing else, you'll be well on your way to the highest levels of enlightenment.*

To begin, Dr. Hawkins gives us a frame of reference as to the history of our country's calibration. He will also address how and why there are dips and raises in these levels of consciousness and what types of things affect them.

I don't know that I can explain the why, other than that's the pattern of the evolution of consciousness on this planet at this time. But we noted that the consciousness level of mankind generally has risen over time. As we learned in Chapter 1, at the time of the birth of the Buddha, the consciousness of mankind overall was 90, and at the time of Jesus's birth, it was up to 100. And during the Middle Ages, it was about 180. It gradually came up to 190. Then the consciousness level of mankind stayed at 190 for many centuries. It didn't change at all. Suddenly, in the year 1988, I think it was, it suddenly jumped from 190 to 205. It not only crossed over 200, it went *beyond* 200. It suddenly jumped and there's no logical explanation for it except maybe that was the destiny of mankind.

I always joke about it. I think, *Well, God probably noticed Earth and had a kindly thought. Bang, it went from 190 to 205.* Or the arch angels said, "What is that crazy planet down there," and had a kindly thought—a loving thought would be sufficient to do it.

I'd say it was the accumulated good karma of mankind—practically speaking, the effort toward goodness, which even though it wasn't instantaneously accomplished, was a design toward goodness—that lifted the level of consciousness.

During World War II, with all the bombing that went on—like the blitz of London, 24 hours a day, month in and month out—most of the great cathedrals escaped unscathed. In 1971, I spoke at some places in Europe, and I noticed how all these buildings survived. Chartres Cathedral in France, and all these other great cathedrals, were somehow spared; mankind on both sides respected what was of great meaning and value. So, it's just an action like that—the decision by both sides to sacrifice gain for the recognition of divinity—that can contribute karmically. We could even calibrate that if we wanted to stop and do research on it. The joint agreement on both sides to spare great cathedrals that go back to antiquity, which took 1,000 years to build, were made for goodness. A massive joint agreement toward some kind of goodness could have a profound influence. It's just like when you raise the level of the sea, you lift all the ships at sea. And what I see mankind generally tries to do is run around from one ship to another and lift first this ship and then that ship, instead of promoting that which would prevail for the common good. That which prevails for the common good would then, of its own goodness, lift everyone up to that level of answerability and responsibility.

The alteration in the level of consciousness is also ascribed to the fact that evolution is not a linear event, that it's like the fermentation process and then it goes quiet for a little bit. It's more like nature where you have a year of great winters and then a year of great summers, and then the various ice ages and all. So, it's more that it's evanescent. I naively thought that once it began going up in the late 1980s, it would continue that way. No, suddenly it took a downturn. It went from 207 down to 204—it's evanescent. It's like a pulse that ebbs and flows. There are periods of great progression, and then there are periods of temporary regression.

But I think the overall destiny of mankind is for consciousness to evolve to the level that physical incarnation is no longer of any particular benefit. I think that 15 percent of the people are above 200, 85 percent are below in the world at large. In America, it's 55 percent are below 200 and I think 45 percent above. So periodically we check the calibration just to see, because you turn on the radio or the television and ask yourself, *Well, how could anybody be attracted to this, or impressed by this, or want to join this, or applaud it, or support it?* Well, if 55 percent of the people are below 200, you can see why that which is sadistic, and lascivious, and dishonest, et cetera, has a very large following.

You can get on a famous television program with a big following and do nothing but spout hatred, paranoid delusions, and conspiracy theories, and rant and rave like a lunatic, and you're going to get a fascinated audience, because for half the people out there, that's where they live: malice, anger, lying, deception.

THE 9 FUNDAMENTALS OF CONSCIOUS SPIRITUAL GROWTH

#1: Developing a sense of truth and integrity

You have to respect truth and integrity. Let's say you're a doctor. You can't go operating on somebody out of an opinion. You've got to have an X-ray; you've got to have a diagnostic test. Your first impression may be completely wrong. You have to be willing to change it. So, you have an obligation that is beyond your own personal opinion. Therefore, to grow spiritually, you have to have respect for the fact that there are many people who have evolved far past where you're at and you respect what they have to say until you can verify it for yourself. So you have to be an expert clinician with yourself and hold off on the final diagnosis until you have all the data in.

I almost died a half-dozen times in my life from the wrong diagnosis. The person had an impression because of what I said in the first paragraph, and it turned out to be completely erroneous. They completely missed the diagnosis. I was in practice for 50 years, and I tell you, you cannot be a successful clinician if you just go with your opinion. You have an inkling when the patient walks in the door, and you could be right 90 percent of the time— but that means 10 percent of the time, you're going to be wrong. So you have to have the humility to realize that your opinions are subject to verification by truth, reality, and facts.

#2: Attaining humility

There's a certain sense you get when you're just being self-servingly narcissistic instead of being clinically detached and really wanting to know what the truth is. If you watch the news, you'll see there's an inclination in your own self to want the story to go in a certain direction: that so-and-so was lying or so-and-so wasn't lying. So, you see that inclination and then you say to yourself, "Where's that inclination coming from? Why would I want to change what the story is to satisfy some opinion I have in myself?" You begin to monitor yourself.

Spirituality is a certain self-awareness and self-monitoring in which you can't just blindly and naively stumble along, falling into this and falling out of that, from one enthusiasm to the next, or one aversion to one attachment. The disciplined spiritual endeavor then is that there is a higher truth, and your dedication is to arrive at it one way or the other. So you ask God to reveal the truth to you. You ask the Holy Spirit for a miracle to allow you to see it as it really is and not as your opinion or your perception is framing it because you begin to realize that your mind makes its selections via framing things, and you frame out what you don't want to have as an option.

Then you reach a certain degree of humility. The essence of spiritual growth is humility that you could be wrong, so you don't have a stake in any outcome, because if you have a stake then it doesn't allow you to learn through experience that you could be wrong. There's an old joke, "I may have a lot of character defects, but being wrong ain't one of them." That's the narcissistic ego speaking.

#3: Self-awareness and self-mastery

This pathway to conscious spiritual growth is through self-awareness. You begin to realize that you're attaching great importance to things out there and that you're projecting value onto them in and of itself. I remember being in London where they have the crown jewels at the Tower of London. I'm standing there looking at the fabulous, wonderful, world-renowned Koh-i-Noor diamond, and it's nothing but a shiny little piece of stone, which would appeal to a child because, of course, it sparkles. When you think of what people went through to get this little glassy sparkle—they're willing to give up empires. The biggest diamond on the planet—there it is and all what people are willing to go through to get it. What would you do with it if you got it? Hide it under your pillow? You couldn't sell it. You couldn't display it.

So you'd get great narcissistic satisfaction out of realizing that you have the most valuable diamond in the world. If somebody finds out you've got it, they'd kill you in an instant, you see, because *they* want the biggest diamond in the world. So the core of narcissism is really pomposity. The pomposity of being right, and the biggest pomposity in today's world is moral superiority.

#4: Accountability

There's an ethical morality, and the basic realization is that you're answerable, and accountable, and responsible. So, if you don't think you're accountable, and you have no responsibility, then you have no ethical obligation, because there is no divinity and there's no one to be accountable to. Strangely, we discovered accidentally that the consciousness calibration technique, which is so simple, was not possible for a good percentage of people. As we mentioned in Chapter 2, an atheist can't use it. People ask, "What's atheism got to do with it?" That which refutes the source and the core of truth is denied the benefit of it. There have been some famous personalities, they're usually professionals who would pooh-pooh the technique and couldn't get it to work. It took me some time to detect what it is and then I finally figured it out. Those who deny the truth of God are denied its benefits. It's not judgmentalism, it's just that the quality of that energy is such that you can't get it to work. Some people just have zero musical talent. They're tone deaf. They can't tell one tone from another on a scale. And then there are other people who are gifted and can tell if you are a quarter tone off. You either have the gift of musicality or you don't have the gift of musicality, and it's probably karmically determined. If you've cursed God and denied God, you can't really expect to get the truth of God at the flick of a switch. You may have to earn it back. So, I think spiritual progress is earned.

Accountability is responsibility, and this is really central to all spiritual evolution. You're either accountable for your answers or you're not. If you consider yourself not accountable, you cannot do the muscle test for truth. If you're not accountable, that negates the value of truth. So those who negate the truth cannot do the test. People below 200 are unable to do it. At the mid-400s is where people are intelligent, integrous, accountable, take responsibility, and are consciously evolving. So, accountability then is necessary.

We realize there are two major classifications of falsehood. The satanic, which is basically evil, violence, et cetera, and the Luciferic, which is the substitution of falsehood for truth. Those that are most evil demonstrate both. They reverse truth to begin with and then have a satanic depiction of God. So, how could it be so prevalent? The Native American Indians saw God as the divinity of nature. But the story of God the great punisher is prevalent, with God depicted in anthropomorphic terms, vengeful and angry. This makes a lot of people turn away from religion. They don't want to face a God that's as bad as a human being. We all have jealousy, anger, and vengefulness, so how do you get to be God with the same character traits?

Then it dawned on me, and I thought, *Why is such a negative depiction of God recurring over millennia and in different parts of the world?* It's because of natural disasters. Earthquakes, and floods, and fire—that's how the gods must be angry. The big mine collapses and there are earthquakes and tsunamis and great plagues. The gods must be angry. That's all it is, isn't it? You have a natural human disaster. The whole principle of karma. You say, "How can that be? How can that be?" There's no explaining it logically why you happened to be there at the time of the tsunami or the earthquake or the flood, why you were in San Francisco during the great earthquake. The angry God would be the obvious conclusion and now you're going to try to assuage this God. You can please him by killing all infidels. Therefore, you see, the negative arises from man's experience and a primitive interpretation based on natural disasters. We have to please this angry God so that he doesn't strike us dead.

We share the fate of mankind, and that's one thing that instead of being divisive can bond us together—that like ourselves, the people who we view as enemies are subject to the same vicissitudes. Accountability and responsibility are critical.

#5: Simplifying your life

The spiritual pathway is not a straight-and-narrow, cut-and-dried pathway at all. It's very erratic. There are periods of great intense spiritual passion and devotion, and in those states you're willing to sacrifice anything, and then there are periods of dryness where nothing seems to be going on. The great saints, of course, in their autobiographies wrote that there are periods when spiritual change is so rapid you're barely able to keep up with it: it's a whole new paradigm of reality replaced by a greater paradigm, replaced by a greater paradigm.

Then there are periods of spiritual dryness. The great saint, Mother Teresa, spoke of these. I contextualized them as periods of dryness, because in a certain state of consciousness, the presence of the divinity of Christ is apparent, but then in another period, you're getting dependent on that and you have to discover the divinity within yourself and not be hanging on just waiting to be inspired by spiritual visions. It's very nice to have the spiritual visions of saints and divinities visiting you, but then at a certain level you have to give up your dependence on that, because there's still an out-there-ness about it. The spiritual vision is still an out-there-ness. And the realization of the Self with a capital *S* is not an out-there-ness; it's an *allness* of the reality of the totality. Periods of great excitement, I've been through all of them. I've been through periods of great drivenness, periods of great ecstasy, periods of enormous calm. *Satchitananda*, that's 600. I remember when I hit that. At that point, you have permission to leave the world. I remember sitting on a rock. I went into the divine state, and I had invitational permission to leave. I could either leave or not leave, because there was no real purpose of maintaining physicality. I wasn't driven in that direction. On the other hand, there wasn't any gain in leaving the physicality. There was neither loss nor gain no matter which way I went. It didn't really matter, so I thought, *Well, I'll just leave things as they are and not really care about it*, and eventually after a number of hours, the body got up and walked away, and that's the way it was.

It's both a choice and a natural state. Each of those states may be sequential or they may alternate at various periods of life. There's a time of spiritual learning. You read all the books, you go to all the lectures, et cetera. You're in acquisition of knowledge and understanding.

Then there are quiet periods when you may withdraw from the world for 10 years and move out of New York City and move out to the sticks to a little town nobody ever heard of and not watch television. For years, I never read the newspaper or a magazine. I had no idea what was going on in the world. I didn't own a television set. If I'd owned one, I wouldn't have turned it on anyway. So that was, let's say, a decade of detachment from the world. You know, I went to town one time and went into a coffee shop and I heard that President Reagan had been shot. I hadn't heard. I had no radio, no television. I wasn't talking with other people, and I was living a very simple monastic lifestyle. There was a whole decade of living a monastic lifestyle. I had a can of soda and a piece of cheese in the refrigerator and that was it. I didn't go anywhere, I didn't need anything, and life was complete and total from instant to instant.

In the unenlightened state, life goes from incomplete to complete, then from incomplete to complete. In the enlightened state, life goes from complete, to complete, to complete. Each instant is already complete. To the average person, incomplete means they have to change this, move that, turn the thermostat up. They're constantly going from incomplete to the next moment. So in the state of completion—I can remember when I finally realized it—you're in the middle of a meal and the doorbell rings and it doesn't bother you that you can't finish your meal. You're already complete. You ate half the meal, and you're already complete.

Being incomplete is thinking, *I can't wait 'til I chew this up and swallow it, and then I will be full and then I will do it again.* You go from incomplete to a greater state of completion. Completion is when everything is complete and satisfied at this moment. As I think of it, everything is complete up to this moment. If we stop now, I'm satisfied that everything is complete. I can fall over right now, lie on the floor, and leave. There's no reason not to, except it would be tacky. You'd have to call an ambulance and the whole rigmarole. You don't want to put that on a friend; you know, he's got to call the medics, and get someone to haul the body away. The whole thing's a drag. So you wouldn't want to do that to a friend. If you're out in the middle of the forest all by yourself and don't have anybody else in your life, you could just lie down and leave, and the bacteria will eat you up over time. No rush.

#6: Having a sense of purpose

We contextualize our lives, giving them significance and meaning, and labeling them. The level of the 300s is a very useful and profound level. That's the level of volunteer firemen, policemen, and mega churches. There's enthusiasm: music, cheering, dancing, and clapping. There's a surge of life energy, and when a whole group gets a surge of life energy like that, it's very invigorating and uplifting, and it certainly brings you above level 200. Getting above level 200 is the most significant part. People under 200 get into the enthusiasm, the contagion, and the spiritual energy of a group like that, and it lifts them up, and they say, "Wow! Here I was ridiculing God, Jesus, and spirituality. This is incredible." They experience joy. So, you lift a group like that with enthusiasm and encouragement, lending them strength and their power.

One classic teaching is to stay with holy company. Only when you yourself have evolved to that level, can you maintain that level *without* the holy company. There is a belief in AA, for instance, that says that if you leave the group and stop going to meetings, you relapse because it wasn't your energy, it was the group's energy. The AA group was calibrated at 540. Staying with holy company is another thing you can do to further your spiritual evolution. Holy company gives you the energy, the motivation, and the backing. As you get more spiritually evolved, you don't need it. It isn't just a matter of needing the support; it's a matter of taking advantage of it. Taking advantage of it to avail yourself of holy company, because it's something our society does offer.

Certainly, when you go into a great cathedral, you're instantly brought into a different frame of mind. I've been in great cathedrals in Europe, and I even spent one night meditating in the great pyramids of Egypt. It's the atmosphere that is contributing a certain amount to you, see? Don't just assume it's either you or it's just the pyramid; it's the interaction between you *and* the pyramid. It's the interaction between you and the Cathedral at Chartres. When you walk the labyrinth in the cathedral, you learn how to fall into the state of consciousness of walking the labyrinth without necessarily going through the mechanics of walking through the labyrinth, but you begin to value that energy field of peace and sense of inner presence that arises.

I had to laugh the last time I was in Chartres cathedral; they've got chairs all over the floor so that people don't start walking the labyrinth. You just do it as a meditative style, and in fact you get the same effect if you have a photograph of it and trace the pattern. There's something unique about that design, and the monks discovered over the years that to merely traverse it mentally, even if it's just with a pencil over the design, puts you into a meditative state.

That's a pretty advanced level of consciousness, though. Most people think they're deficient and have to do something special in order to reach that state, and I say, "How can you reach a divine higher state if you've bought it at the cost of the suffering and death of others? I mean, how do you justify karmically that you're going to go to heaven, and the only way you're going to go to heaven is by killing others?" That seems to be very convoluted, or at least it's not aligned with my own understanding of divinity and universal love.

People always say, "What can I do about the world?" Ramana Maharshi says the world you see doesn't even exist. It's actually just your perception of the world. You think the world needs *you*, but it needs you like a hole in the head, actually. Each person's evolution contributes to the level of the sea; each person, by making your life a prayer. When I give sermons occasionally, the sermon is always about converting your life into a prayer. Become that about which you talk and learn and read and sing hymns—become *that*. Because by being that, just your existence already transforms the world. Each one of us raises the level of the sea not by what we do and say, but by what we have become. The great kings and emperors and conquerors have come and gone. They've all come and gone and made all kinds of waves. And what did that do? Nothing. You realize it has nothing to do with your perception, nothing to do with your judgmentalism.

#7: Lovingness

There are various phases where loving others is wonderful, but you don't love yourself. And then there's the narcissistic love for yourself and not others. Then you might give that up, and you love all life and all its expressions. With this lovingness, you see the intrinsic value of all that exists, and you see the divinity of all that exists. The inner source of existence is divinity itself, which is formless, but then it takes form: window, wall, door, tree, microphone, carpet. But it is the nonlinear presence of divinity within that allows for linear existence in the first place. Without divinity as the source of existence, nothing would exist, much less the linear form.

There is a realization then of the divinity of all that exists, including one's own self. There's an obligation to God to become all that you can be, and there's how you serve God: Not by money in the plate, although that's helpful at a certain phase. Not by good works, not by giving to the poor, not by picnics for the handicapped. Your obligation to divinity is to perfect your own self to the greatest degree possible, to be thankful for the gifts, and then to pursue those gifts to see how you can best use them for mankind. I mean in my own life, you see, I was gifted in many ways. It was like a burden, actually. There was a sense of moral obligation, a pressure, which partially led to my becoming a physician. I thought devoting myself to the relief of human suffering was the ultimate calling. Then I saw that suffering on the physical level was bad enough, but on the mental level it was even worse, because at least on the physical level, you could do something tangible. You could operate, give an injection, anesthesia, antibiotics. The suffering within, which was really a state of consciousness, and the relief of human suffering was what I knew I was very attracted to as a physician, psychiatrist, and spiritual teacher. And the motivation that I have now is to share what from the highest level I think relieves human suffering: advancing your own consciousness just by its own nature automatically relieves suffering and increases the level of happiness.

I went from physician, to psychiatrist, to spiritual teacher. And the research that I do is to increase that eventual development. You don't try to change other people. Some people are motivated to change others. If you realize that becoming all that you can be to the best of your capacity fulfills your obligation, then the consequences of that are no longer in your hands—they're up to divinity.

#8: Overcoming the darkness

Hatred is infectious, and a lynch mob demonstrates it. Look at what happened after the Civil War among the various sections of society, the Ku Klux Klan, and all the various political groups that circulated. Mankind is constantly evolving, and it does so in an irregular, fragmented fashion. A path that leads one person down a bad road is uplifting to another, and it depends on what your motivation is to walk that path and what your level of consciousness was at the time. Your need to understand purpose and your goal, and to own the downside of yourself.

The levels of consciousness are calibrated from 200 up, and then there's 200 down. To transcend them, you then have to own them without going into moralistic judgmentalism. For one thing, each negative feeling is not by itself. All the negative feelings occur at the same time, actually. The one most prominent at times may be anger, but underneath the anger was envy, and underneath the envy was a feeling of being depressed, and underneath feeling depressed was resentment. And so this shadow would be just the whole collective, everything that calibrates below 200.

Now most people with spiritual honesty admit when they're annoyed, admit when they're angry, admit when they feel guilty, and they explore it. They explore to see where that leads, and where that arises from. And you discover that each negative feeling is stacked upon the one below it. You're prideful. Why are you prideful? Because you feel deficient. Why do you feel deficient? Because your wantingness is not satisfied. And why is your wantingness not satisfied? Because you're angry. And why are you angry? The shadow is really the collective. All of them usually happen at the same time. You're angry—why are you angry? Because somebody hurt your pride. Pride is egotism inflated.

Your problem is not that you think too little of yourself, but that you think too much of yourself. The world should cater to you. Your indignation, and your anger, and your pride, and your resentment all collect together. Eventually they all end up at the bottom, which is hopelessness and despair, when you give up all together and just rock back and forth in your chair and say, "There's nothing I can do about it. I'm a hopeless failure."

It's the hated enemy that is the projection of their own dark side. They see the Communist as the ultimate evil, or the fascists, or the Republicans, or the Democrats, or Blacks, or women. There's racism, sexism, religionism, ageism.

• • •

I've told you about my own inner experiences of letting go and surrendering everything until I came to and there was nothing left to surrender to God and everything was silent. And then came the awareness out of nowhere—I had not surrendered my life to God. I had surrendered everything else, but not life. And then came the knowingness that this too must be surrendered. I'd surrendered joy, ecstasy, peace, serenity, all kinds of things to God. All was gone and all was silent. I was in a very high space. There was no one there, no other entities.

In the high spaces there are no other entities talking to you or giving you instructions or giving you dictations. Nothing but the knowingness that came out of nowhere, the knowingness that that which I am is beyond life and death. Clinging to life was the last thing. The tenacity of hanging on to life. I surrendered life. "All fear is illusion," came the knowingness.

The voice of the teacher that radiates forth from the aura has to come from absolutism. It cannot come from relativism or thinkingism. It has to come from the absolutism of absolute knowingness of having been there and done that. So the absolutism of the knowingness was that I would surrender this to God. I surrendered life itself. Lifetime after lifetime you don't surrender the source of life itself, because this is the very core of the narcissistic ego that thinks it is the author of life, the center and the core of life. In surrendering what the mind has believed for eons, up came a great terror. It was a severe terror, and fortunately, it only lasted for a few moments.

If you surrender to the terror, the terror disappears and the fear is gone forever. The fear, which had been there forever, is now gone forever. The mortality, then, is first the mortality of the physicality, of this particular incarnation. And eventually as you keep letting go of things, the fears all disappear. Whatever happens to you is irrelevant. Why is it irrelevant? Because it's God's problem. If the ceiling falls on us all now, it's God's problem, isn't it? We're just going to sit and wait and see what God's going to do about it. Maybe he'll get a truck or a derrick here, or ambulances, and maybe he won't. Maybe you'll breathe; maybe you won't.

What happens then is you need to come back to this particular life again, with the acceptance of mortality as an inevitability and get over the fear of it. And it is only a matter of acceptance. The fear of death is what makes this seem awful, because you're struggling with it. Once you accept it, it's not awful at all. You die . . . so what? Big deal. It's okay.

One reason people have a fear of dying is because of moral accountability. The reason they don't want to die is because they know they're going to be faced with it. Seeing yourself as you really are, you think, *I don't want that to be on my soul forever. I don't want that. I don't want that unkindness. I don't want that negativity. I don't want that selfishness to be there, and I beg for a chance to correct that.* Then, you're going to be more sympathetic, more understanding, more forgiving, more loving. You're going to value life above winning. Moral accountability is why most people are afraid to die, because you realize that you're about to get confronted with the truth of what you have been. If we accept moral accountability as we go through life, we don't build up a fear about it.

Of course, at this point you see your beliefs of divinity come forth as part of your moral accountability and part of your fear of death. As you grow spiritually you can see that the fear of death lessens, because you picture God as merciful. You realize on your deathbed you're going to have a companion.

The concept of divinity is merciful or punitive. The depths of hell is not something anyone wants to experience, even for a few seconds. Besides, you can't experience it for a few seconds, because each second is experientially an eternity. So, in choosing between heaven and hell, one decision takes you closer to heaven and the next decision takes you closer to hell. If you become spiritually very advanced, you realize that it's not worth taking the chance. There's a temporary gain to vanity, and controlling others, and getting revenge. There's a short chuckle as you punch somebody in the face. Maybe they deserved it. However, moral accountability then takes you to a choice between two doors. One door leads to heaven and the other door leads to hell.

God does not throw you into hell; you yourself by your own choices have brought you to that state of abject despair and hopelessness. What are the limits of freedom? Frankly, there aren't any, are there? There aren't any limits to freedom. You can choose to hate God. You can choose to love God. You can choose to be generous. You can choose to be stingy. What are the limits of freedom? Only the capacity of the human mind to see what the options are—the willingness to see the options, whether you're grasping or generous, flexible, and able to learn, grow, mature. Most people say, "Well, I think what I'll do is I'll try to learn from this experience. I'll try and make every part of my life about growing and maturing, and developing spiritually." There's an innate energy to life. It's called élan vital, and that's a French term meaning one's life energy. The energy flows through you as a certain energy. Life flows as an energy.

You can look at it theologically as a reality. We know that the calibrated levels of consciousness go all the way to 1,000, and what the world calls evil is below 200. There are TV programs where everybody applauds the negativity. The host is overtly pouring forth hatred, conspiracy theories. Now, where do they get such an audience? Would a group of spiritually evolved people be interested in watching conspiracy theories spit out with contempt, anger, and hatred? How much appeal would it have in heaven? It would have a big audience in hell. Killing, murder, and torture are not very appealing as you spiritually evolve, and when it comes on screen, you say, "Good God, what do I want to watch that for?"

#9: Developing a sense of humor

You begin to see that humor serves mankind to a greater degree than the people leading the parade. All the great enthusiasm—save the planet, and save the world, and all that stuff—making a big, ostentatious display of it all. Actually, a good sense of humor to me is more spiritually evolved than all that pious, holier-than-thou do-goodism.

Humor recontextualizes things. It puts it in a different context. And humor arises out of the contrast between the linear content and the nonlinear context, which is what makes it humorous. And the great humorists live long. People like Jack Benny or George Burns. George Burns made it to 100. Half the time they fall over in the bathtub and die of a fractured skull. I'm reminding myself, when I get to be their age—do not take showers in the bathtub.

CONSCIOUS SPIRITUAL GROWTH

I think Ronald Reagan demonstrated the characteristics of conscious spiritual growth. He calibrated like 500 or something. Winston Churchill, too; he single-handedly held together the British empire in its darkest day. Churchill calibrated over 500. He was the heart of the lion; he stood up and got the British people to face the blitz.

The rallying call can come from people with greatness of heart, and Churchill had that. There are scientists who had greatness of spirit, like Louis Pasteur. They got ridiculed for the advances they made. Greatness of spirit means even though you know you're going to be criticized, you see the great benefit. Some people believed bacteria caused infection, and they almost got killed for believing it. But because of it, we have the discovery of antibiotics and other life-saving innovations. Anything that relieves human suffering and furthers the evolution of consciousness is of great value. Some people spearhead it and contribute by their endorsement of it. These great philanthropic organizations uplift others by promoting education and health.

How can we help others? First, you fulfill what you can, and then you reach the point where you become philanthropic, not necessarily financially, but philanthropic as a state of consciousness. You ask yourself, *What do I want from the world right now?* Nothing. Then, *What do I do with my life?* Because most people spend their whole lives chasing their wants, their desires. Well, what happens then, when you have them all? What happens when you've fulfilled all your desires? Does your life then become worthless? No. Because you share what you have become with others. You share what you have become.

The ultimate act of lovingness is to share that which you have become, so that your life becomes a prayer. You become that which you preach and teach. You hold with love, you hold with respect, you hold the world together in a way within your arms of love.

Close your eyes now and picture the whole world and the whole population of the world. Open your heart and radiate that light to the world and embrace it. Let's all put our arms around this whole world, every living thing on the world, every little toad, every kangaroo, every person, and put our arms around it and radiate that love and uplift the love by our intention. By becoming infinitely loving, we become the destiny of mankind, which is the realization of divinity within as the source of one's existence.

In the beginning, people learn. They have to, otherwise they don't even know it's possible. Then after a while, learning gets in the way because they get caught up in belief systems instead of realizing the truth of it experientially. To learn, in the beginning, is to get oriented to the subject; then you pick what seems comfortable and useful in your life, and you pursue that. And then at a certain point you stop reading about it. I've given my own spiritual library away several times in my lifetime. You accumulate a couple hundred books and then you say, "This is all mentalism and linearity," and you give it all away. Then another decade or two later, you start accumulating the books all over again. Then you clear them all out again.

THE GREATEST MISCONCEPTION
ABOUT SPIRITUAL GROWTH

People think spiritual growth is going to involve sacrifice, but it doesn't. You sacrifice the negatives, and some people would consider that a sacrifice, I suppose. There's time and energy, and if you've got a family, you may wonder where do you get the time and the energy? There are certain periods of life when you've got a young, growing family and you're trying to make it in the world, and this is not usually the best time to decide you're going to become a monk.

You can make a lifestyle change perhaps later in life. I think a lot of people look forward to getting older, when they will have what's needed to spend more time on spiritual life. In many churches you'll see the congregation is primarily older. There will be some young people with children, yes, but you'll see that well over half the congregation is gray haired (in some churches maybe 80 percent gray and white hair). Cynics might say, "Well they're just afraid of dying, that's all." No, it's because they've finally got enough space in their lives and the leisure to do it. They now have the time and the energy and the spiritual interest to improve their lives. Young people say, "I haven't got time for this." Well, wait until a later time. Or learn to do spiritual work in small bits, in snippets. Five minutes of friendliness. I say the best thing to do is to be friendly to everybody and loving toward everybody.

Every clerk in the store, I always thank them, and people will just practically faint. Try it with every clerk in every store and every person you run into—just be as smiling and loving toward them as you can be. It just bowls them over. They just look at you like, "Huh? What?"

I did this for years in New York City. I would walk by an apartment building on Fifth Avenue, past the doormen, and I would say good morning to them all and smile. Pretty soon, they looked forward to it, and I discovered that one can smile and stop and say hello to anybody. I can walk down any New York City street and strike up a conversation with almost anybody almost instantly. Because of your openness and your lovingness, they don't feel danger or fear. The animal instinct in them perceives that you're a safe space.

As your consciousness evolves, people treat you differently. They look forward to seeing you; they feel uplifted by your presence. If you attend the party, it's a success. Just your energy radiates around the whole room. You serve others by what you have become. The more loving you become, the more you're serving your fellow man and serving God.

Chapter 8

SPIRITUAL PRACTICES

Now that you have the fundamentals of conscious spiritual growth in place, you need to begin a program of regular spiritual practices to keep you in spiritual shape and help you deepen your sense of spiritual awareness.

In this enlightening chapter, Dr. Hawkins will describe some of the most important and effective spiritual practices he recommends, from the most basic practices to the most advanced.

MEDITATION

The meditative practice deepens your understanding of any religion, much like contemplation. What I usually emphasize is both meditation and aligning your life so that you make your life the prayer. You try to live and become that which you are studying and learning. You become forgiving. In the beginning, forgivingness seems like an artificial practice. Jesus Christ said, "Forgive them, for they know not what they do." That's a mentalization, and when you're angry at somebody, it may cross your mind, and you think, *Well, I should probably be seeing it differently, but I don't.* But as you get deeper in it, then you think, *Well, how can I see this through different eyes? How can I alter my experience of this?* Then that requires a deeper study. You're trying to go from the familiarity of the intellectual to the experiential. You're trying to become that which was formerly mental and is now incorporated into your personality and your way of actually being in the world.

Meditation, of course, has a great history and we could spend hours just describing all the meditative pathways. I've experimented and tried them all. I belonged to the First Zen Institute in New York City back in the '50s, and I practiced Zen meditation for many years. For over 20 years, I meditated an hour in the morning and an hour in the afternoon. You meditate on some specific truth that you've picked up until you really become the awareness of the truth and the reality of that. Then you don't need to tell yourself, "Well, I should be forgiving that person." You start to see, eventually, that everybody is only being what they are, what they can be at the moment. Everybody is just being what they could be at the moment, and if not, it's because they can't be. If they were able to be different, they would be. You have a certain sympathy for everyone, that everyone is pretty much stuck with the human condition. And the human condition is, frankly, extremely difficult, for the individual as well as for whole societies and civilizations.

The thing about meditation is it takes you away from the world. In other words, you've got to set aside an hour in the morning and an hour in the afternoon or at night, like I did. And what happens to a lot of people is they compartmentalize it. When they're meditating, that's one thing, and then they go back into the world, and that's another thing. People do that with religion, too, of course. On Sunday, they're very religious and then Monday, they're back to their usual business, padding the bill as usual but maybe feeling a little guilty about it. But it gets compartmentalized.

After a while, many people give up meditation because it interferes with daily life. They're too busy this morning, so they skip it, and then tomorrow's too busy, too. Meditation then tends to get lost. Contemplation is a lifestyle of sharpened awareness. The nearest classic teaching of it is mindfulness. Mindfulness is to always be aware, to be consciously aware of what your mind is doing at all times, to not go unconscious and become oblivious to your own inner mental workings. You become familiar with the mind. By becoming familiar, the mind actually changes as you become more and more familiar with it.

A contemplative lifestyle is more effective. It's a way of being in the world, because now you're trying to *become* that which you have studied. You can do it continuously. A person can be contemplative no matter what they're doing. My own lifestyle was contemplative for many years, and I was aware of exactly how I was being with each specific incident. That way, you become more aware of the reality of other people, as well. You become aware of their reality, and get out of the solipsistic view that reality is how *you* see it. You become aware that there's a reality, and this is just the way you are seeing it. This is not the way the world is—it's the way you're seeing the world.

A sudden understanding of that came relatively early in my life, when I was on all kinds of big talk shows in New York City. When you go to these places, because you're the celebrity of the day, everybody flatters you and they take you into the makeup room and you get all made up. You're the star of the moment. The TV show starts, and there are millions of people watching you. But, when the show ends, all the lights go out, the hundreds of people in the studio disappear, and you can hear almost an echo. You leave the building, and there you are, out on the street, and suddenly there is a sinking feeling. I understand why rock stars and celebrities do drugs, because when the show is over, you can't handle going from that high to a crash to nothing. I have a sympathy for them.

With meditation, in the beginning at least, you can go into states of samadhi, very high states, and in the beginning the state only lasts while you're *in* that state, while your eyes are closed and you're sitting cross-legged and breathing, and all such, and that marvelous state comes. But then as you get up and walk around, it disappears. Then, as spiritual evolution progresses, the state continues.

In the next stage, it continues even when you open your eyes, and then when you get up and walk around, it disappears. But then the state gets more and more prevailing, and you can get up and walk around in that state, and it remains. Then eventually, you can continue a relatively normal life and the condition is permanent. Eventually, the state precludes what you would call ordinary mentalization all together and you more or less stay in the state. Then the state eventually prevails, and you leave the world, which is what I did. You didn't have any choice; you left the world.

And then after some years, one learns how to reaccommodate the world. It took me many years to learn how to become functional within the world again. It's a completely different nature. It's something that you witness. Just as I'm talking to you now, there's an aspect that witnesses this as a phenomenon that is occurring of its own. It doesn't have anything to do with a personal *I* or *me*. It happens autonomously, just like the bird flies through the air. It happens of its own, and it becomes what I call the persona. There's an interactive energy between the world and the Self with a capital *S* that learns how to re-function in the world.

Most people when they reach an extremely high level of consciousness do not return to the world. They do not function in the world. It's really quite statistically unusual to do so, in fact. Most people stay in a permanent retreat, or they live in an ashram, and if you want to see them, you travel many miles and they smile at you sweetly and bless you and then that's it.

By the grace of God, my capability to explain things and teach returned, so I accepted that was the case, and therefore, I continued to teach. But at the time, because of the extreme nature of the change of consciousness, there wasn't any choice but to leave the world. Its values had no more attraction. There was no point to persevere in that, and also, one has an intuitive knowingness that something else quite different is being called for, so I more or less walked away from everything that the world cherishes as the ultimate.

When you reach this state, you just witness the transition and the changes. People worry about what will happen to them if they reach a certain state where they can't function in the world, so I tell them, "Well, at that state, you *can't* function in the world." The thing is, when that state arises, you're no longer afraid of it. It's just like your hair turning gray; it's not exactly scary. It's just what it is.

• • •

There's a certain point where you're satisfied with what you can do in the world, and you can see that if you keep doing it, it's just more, but it's more of the same. After you have enough millions, what are you going to do with an extra million? It's just a nuisance, you know? You have to call an accountant and say, "Look, I got an extra five million from the company. Figure out what to do with it, okay?" And you hang up. There's no interest.

Pursuing success within the world loses its meaning once you've achieved it, and you know that you've achieved it. Now, a person who you might say is karmically destined to evolve will first satisfy himself. They have satisfied everything that they want from the world, and then they look for something beyond, and they find that they are attracted to spiritual work. A certain number of people are attracted once they've reached success. There are many people, of course, who are highly attracted along the way. They don't wait that many years to feel they've mastered the world before they decide to leave it. They just leave it because the spiritual motivation is strong.

People have karmic propensity, strong karmic propensities. Some people have powerful spiritual drives from early life, but then the person turns away from the world and now finds a whole new area of interest. It's like being reborn. It's a new life. Some people would call it being reborn, being awakened to the spiritual reality and a whole new dimension and meaning to existence. And then rarely, one in 10 million will decide they are attracted to the whole pathway to enlightenment and decide they will make whatever decisions they have to in their life to facilitate that. They may join an ashram. Certainly, they begin to meditate on a very regular, major basis.

When I first came out to a small town, I spent the entire day in a meditative state. I'd start to meditate at 7:00 in the morning. It was just a total change of lifestyle. But I always tell people, you don't have to worry about it, because it won't happen until you're ready for it. You're not going to be suddenly jerked out of your desk at your office and forced to join an ashram. More likely, it's as if you've had enough chocolate and now you want to move on to vanilla. You've satiated that desiringness. You're giving up your addiction to the world when you hit bottom.

For people who are addicted to the world and the novelty of the world and the entertainment of the world, if they keep doing spiritual work, eventually and suddenly, they get released from that addiction. The real addiction, of course, is to the ego's experiencing of the world. Remember, it's not the world. It's your *experience* of the world. So, there's something about the way you're experiencing the world that you now have become addicted to. And if you focus there, then you really start to make fast progress.

You realize you're not addicted to the world, you're addicted to what you get out of it. You begin to look at how the ego is juicing every experience. What is it getting out of these experiences? And then you begin surrendering that to God. So you don't have to surrender the Cadillac, what you surrender is the feeling of pride and success and the narcissistic satisfaction of owning that Cadillac.

With spiritual progression, you begin to appreciate simplicity, and the simpler things are, the better they are.

CONTEMPLATION

There's meditation and then there's contemplation. I favor contemplation because contemplation is a way of being in the world. To make your life appear is a form of contemplation. Contemplation is a way in which you align yourself with context instead of content; with context and intention that your life is of service to the Lord and to your fellow human being, and out of unconditional love, you ask God to transform how you understand the world. It's a way of being in the world, and it's contextualizing the meaning, significance, and intention of your life. That recontextualization then transforms perception, and how you see things differs from the way the world sees them.

The mind looks out and it sees form. That's the linear. The mind registers that and it recognizes it. How does it do this? It does it because the mind is always watching. At first you think you're the content, that you're linear and restricted. This registers, and it's recognition, but how do you know what's going out? Here's the first jump you can make. You can realize that you are not the *content* of what is being witnessed. You think, *I am the witnesser. I am the watcher, the experiencer, the observer witness.* If you have a contemplative lifestyle, it's very easy to recognize. You don't have to meditate, do a lot of weird breathing and stuff. Pranayama breathing, by the way, calibrates at 190. That's the hard way to get there. It takes a lot of Kleenex because of all of the sniffling.

I don't believe in artificial means of energy manipulation. There are many techniques out there that are sold for a price. *"Secrets of the ancient mystics . . . for only $5,000, I'll tell you what they are."* By intention, it's very simple to see that the reason you know what's going on is because there is a watchingness and an experiencingness and this phenomena is happening spontaneously. There's no you that's watching or experiencing. That's a conclusion. Watching and experiencing and awareness, the observing and the witnessing, is happening autonomously.

When you move from identifying with "out there," you realize that consciousness is observing and witnessing all the time, and this phenomena is autonomous. There's no you deciding to be aware. Awareness is happening of its own accord. It's a phenomenon that's intrinsic to your existence. The light of consciousness is intrinsic to your existence. It's not volitional. You withdraw from out-there-ness and you begin to see everything is occurring spontaneously on its own because of its own potential actualizing.

The potentiality actualizes spontaneously. There is no you that thinks about it and decides to do it and then takes the credit or blame for having had it happen. You begin to realize that being aware itself is spontaneous, autonomous, and non-volitional. Behind the light of consciousness, you then begin to realize the self, and out of that, the awareness that even the self is spontaneously being what it is. There's no *you* involved in all of it, so there's no personal you involved in anything about your life at all. It's all delusional. Isn't that nice?

I think intention is what sets karmic patterns. Because actions are pretty autonomous. I mean, what you're taking responsibility for is the intention. There's a famous saying used in 12-Step groups: you're responsible for the effort and not the result. You're karmically accountable for your intention, but the consequences of the action are up to God and the whole universe, and the world the way it is. Intention sets your karmic pattern, and it's your culpability. You can make a big mistake out of innocence and although you're accountable, you're not severely culpable. You can make very serious errors and be extremely culpable for things that are really vicious by intention. You see it all the time, with certain websites and blogs. The intention of these sites is to injure and hurt another person. Even if they feign innocence and have some excuse, nevertheless, the intention is quite glaringly obvious, which is to personally injure a person and insult and denigrate them. If you do that, then you have the karmic consequence of intending to harm another person out of malice. You can try to veil it with some pseudo-sophisticated sophistry, but the intention is pretty clear and obvious.

As you evolve, spiritually you become more and more aware of essence and you become more difficult to fool. People are more difficult to fool as they sharpen their awareness.

PRACTICAL STEPS FOR A MEDITATION PRACTICE

Meditation, of course, has a great history going back thousands of years, and almost everybody does it in either a Hindu or Buddhic style. Meditation is a part of Christianity too, but it is not stylized like it is in Eastern religions. I tell people the simpler you can make it, the better. You just sit quietly and close your eyes. Now if you do that, and you look straight ahead, you'll notice it's not only just dark, but there are tiny, dancing little pinpoints of light. Those are called phosphenes, and you just stare straight ahead.

Now some people recommend concentrating on the breath. To me, that's even too complicated, but if you like you can become aware of the breath. Then, what you do is become the witness of the phenomena that arise within the mind. You don't try to do anything about it. You don't try to suppress thought. You become a witness of that which parades across the mental land-scape. You begin to study with constant focus. You become aware that thoughts are not following each other. The sequence is one of witnessing. Actually, thoughts are coming out of nothingness. People say, "I can't meditate because there are all these thoughts," and they try to stop thoughts. That's a waste of time. You cannot stop thoughts.

There's a certain spiritual belief system that there is a space between two thoughts, and you will glimpse eternity between two thoughts. Well, I tell you, you will not glimpse eternity between two thoughts. I've asked many large congregations of people, "Has anybody every succeeded?" And nobody ever has, because that's not where the blankness is. The blankness is *below* the thoughts. It's prior to the thoughts. The thoughts follow each other in 1/10,000th of a second. Now, the experiencer, the perceiver aspect of the experiencer function of the ego, can't operate that fast. Therefore, you're trying the impossible. You're trying to see something that occurs in less than 1/10,000th of a second, and the detector of this doesn't operate that fast. You'll never find a blank space between two thoughts.

What's happening is the thoughts are like flying fish coming out of the ocean. As you see each flying fish, you notice that this fish over here is not causing that fish over there. So, you don't look to the flying fish; the thoughts have occurred already. What you look to is the ocean. You look *below* thoughts. The place to look for the infinite silent space is below thoughts. If you look at thoughts as a field on the horizon, now you look below the thoughts and you will see that each thought is arising separately, individually, autonomously out of an infinite field of silence, and even as you read these words right now, you think that your mind is busy reading but underneath that is an infinite silence. If it wasn't for that infinite silence, you wouldn't be able to read nor discern the meaning of the words nor detect the languaging. It's because of the infinite silence of the mind.

For this same reason, when you're out in the woods, you wouldn't be able to hear a bird if it wasn't for the infinite silence.

Without the infinite silence in the background, you would not be able to hear anything. The bird's song is not interfering with the silence, it's occurring *within* the silence, and therefore, you approach the mind with the same understanding. Because of the silence, you're aware of what you're thinking and feeling. Look to the silence. When you look at a room, it's because of the emptiness of the room that you can see the furniture. You begin to function closer to that which you are. Ever, ever closer is the infinite silence itself, because that's the silence of the field of consciousness itself. The reason these discussions about science and consciousness go nowhere is because they constantly ruminate about intellectualizations about the *content* of consciousness.

Consciousness is the field itself. It's the field itself in which the thinkingness and all goes on. Consciousness is infinite and it's formless. It's outside of time and space. That's why with consciousness research, using a simple kinesiologic question and answer, you can discern anything that ever happened anywhere in time or space. Everything that happens is recorded within this infinite field of consciousness forever. For eternity. Everything, every thought, feeling, deed, everything you've ever said is recorded forever.

That is the foundation and the basis of karma. Karma means by intention, every action has now imprinted forever in the field of consciousness itself. One, therefore, is accountable for that which you have chosen to become.

What happens to you then is merely the consequence of your own choices. There is no arbitrary god sitting up there as a big horrible judge that's going to throw you in hell if he's mad at you or favor you and have the rain fall on you in great years of prosperity. That's primitive, mythical, cultural, but not really the way it looks when you examine it up close. Divinity is impartial. By virtue of what it is, all things sort themselves out by virtue of that which they have become. And that which they have become, they have become via their own options and decisions. So to be responsible means to be aware of that. Do you want the karma of doing that? Don't ask yourself, *Do I want to do that?* Ask yourself, *Do I want the karma of doing that?* Then you see you have responsibilities.

You could weigh options by saying, "Which karmic consequence would I like?" When you look at it from that viewpoint, it's a lot easier to make moral decisions. What do I want to have to live with, for God knows how long (in eternity, even)? As I talk about accountability and culpability versus responsibility, it becomes clear that you're responsible, and then the degree of morality is a whole different understanding. People mix up the two, but you can innocently make a mistake. It's always the *intention* of the action. Wisdom evolves slowly.

PSYCHOLOGICAL MEDITATION

With psychological meditation, there are usually trainings. They'll give you a mantra to repeat or a divine image to hold in mind, or a combination, and certain postures and breathing styles. You might say that's the formal mechanics. That's the content of the meditative style: how you sit, how you breathe, which mantra and symbols you use, et cetera. That's one style. Then you begin to witness. You try to move to the witness/observer. You begin to witness the phenomena of the mind as they rebuild themselves without doing anything about them. At that point, as I mentioned briefly before, you go past the form of the thoughts themselves and you find the infinite silent space. The infinite silent space then leads you to what is the infinite silent space and the awareness of consciousness itself, which is intrinsically without content.

And, how does one know that the silent space is there? It's because of awareness. One becomes aware of an infinite silence that is below and more universal than the content of the mind, and then one starts trying to move into the source, the very source of that consciousness awareness. The source of the consciousness awareness leads you to the pronoun *I*. Then comes the unveiling of the fact there is no such entity and as you look for the personal I, no such thing exists. You come to a final definition of the I when you've let go of all of the descriptions, all the adjectives and the adverbs. The I is not doing anything, and one comes to the source of this sense of I, and one comes to the awareness that I is the source of life, that I and life are united.

That leads you to very advanced states, including the abandonment of even life itself to God. The abandonment of self as the very source of life created an agonizing experience of death. On the other side of that door stood the glory and infinite reality out of which emerges all of the universe as a continual emergence, which we call life; but that's the *appearance* of life. That's not life itself. One confuses the appearance of life with the *source* of life. The source of life is invisible. The appearance of life is transitory so you can't get attached to the transitory appearance. Instead, you constantly look within.

The source of life is invisible.

The phenomena are all happening of their own. The talkingness is happening of its own, and your questioning this is happening spontaneous and autonomously. The two of us are here together, due to our joint karmic inheritance and that of the whole world. In fact, all eternity has occurred up to this very moment. This is the emergence of the future that we're sitting on. We're sitting on the disappearing edge of the past and the advancing age of the future, so if we're clever, we'll stay put and avoid both of them. Reality is not aligned with either one. It transcends them. It transcends time. Even once you're aware of that—that what is speaking now is not even occurring in time, that time is something that you project onto things, and that time and space and location are all projections of the human consciousness—you won't bypass the mind when you first start meditating, because what you're confronted with is the traffic on the street and the sounds and the thoughts going and the feeling and the itch in your foot and all these things. You're not going to bypass that because bypassing it is pretty late stage, to be independent of the content of the mind. Eventually, the mind stops and becomes silent. It's a great relief.

There are different stages. They're not different styles; they're really a stage. Even when you get to advanced stages of meditation, when you first sit down, the mind is still talking, but now you've learned quickly how to bypass it. You go through the stages much more quickly. Also, there's certain visual phenomena. It's like the inside of your mind lights up and there's a certain sequence to that. I can remember there was a meditation group I went to one time many years ago, and there was a certain stage we called the Bright Blue after you'd been meditating a certain number of minutes. It's like all of a sudden everything within the mind is lit up in a rather intense blue.

The deeper stages were beyond the Bright Blue, but the Bright Blue told you that you were entering a deeper meditation. You're going into deeper and deeper layers of the mind, of the unconscious, of the spirit of consciousness. Deeper and deeper levels, and at each one, you say, "This must be the ultimate." It's like a door opens. This must be the ultimate, but beyond the ultimate is another ultimate and beyond that ultimate is another ultimate. And that's how you get really intrigued with meditation, because just as you escape one level to a state of even greater ecstasy, joy, and awareness, there is yet another stage beyond that, and yet another, and yet another, and you see what it is that's holding you back from yet another. Let's say, for example, you can get attached to familiarity. You say, "Oh, I can see. I'm attached to 'this is the way it's going to be.'"

The Bright Blue is very intriguing and then you got to let go of being hooked on the Bright Blue and let it be of its own.

CONTEMPLATION PRACTICES

Contemplation is continuous. It's like you're constantly paying attention to one thing. Let's say that your assignment for the day is to become aware of the intrinsic perfection and beauty of all that exists, the holiness and the sacredness of all of creation. Wow. That'll keep you busy for the next 20, 30 years! But in the orientation, you say, "Dear God, I'm trying to see the perfection and beauty of all of existence and I ask for thy blessing." There's supplication to God to help you on this trip, and then you've stated your intention. Your intention is to go beyond the linear, beyond perception, beyond your thoughts, opinions, and all of that narcissistic stuff about the world, and see the world as it exists. You're going past differentiation between perception and essence.

What you're really asking in meditation and contemplation is to go beyond duality, to stop interpreting perception as reality. Instead, to sense the essence of things, to sense the exquisite. For instance, this morning I walked around and it was still dark, and suddenly in the darkness, I heard this loud purr. And that was my white kitty, picking up the energy of that which I am. When I pick up his energy, the interaction of those two energies sends us both into a state of bliss, happiness, contentment, and love, with the joyful presence of God. I don't have to do anything within the linear domain except be there. All I have to do is stand there, and the white kitty starts to purr. He purrs because I'm there, because of that which I am. You see, that which the cat is, the cat is a responder to love. In the presence of love, the white kitty automatically starts to purr. In fact, all I have to do is look across the room and think of him, and have a loving thought about him, and it turns him on and he starts to purr. It's just amazing. That's the way the world becomes.

It's just like when people say New York is a cold, unfriendly place, which I mentioned in Chapter 3. Give me a break. I could walk on any street, start talking to anybody about anything, and have an instant friendly conversation strike up, just like we were all friends for hundreds of years.

Meditation and contemplation are very exciting. They're very exciting because the discoveries that you make are amazing. You start looking within for what's exciting in the world and not what's without.

In this next part, Dr. Hawkins takes you into the world of the true mystic. He shares some of the characteristics that you can look for and expect when you seek to discover the enlightened state. He also shares some practical exercises that you can begin to practice that will assist you in the evolution of your consciousness.

THE 9 CENTRAL ELEMENTS OF SERIOUSLY COMMITTED INNER SPIRITUAL WORK

#1: Discipline of focus without deviation.

One-pointedness of mind is a certain style of meditation. You focus on an object, a thought, a feeling, a divine figure, a mantra, or a sound perhaps. With fixity of mind, you keep your focus on it. This takes discipline. The mind wants to wander away, and with the undisciplined mind, passing thoughts run away with the mind. You start by disciplining your mind to concentrate on the point of a pen and to keep it there unwaveringly. Eventually, you can perfect it so that nothing breaks your concentration.

#2: Willingness to surrender all desires and fears to God.

Spiritual awareness is far beyond emotionality. You're willing to surrender the emotion. What you're really surrendering is the payoff of the emotion, because first there is the emotion, then there's what you get out of that emotion. And to let go of emotion, you have to let go of the payoff. People love to be indignant. They love to be the victim. They wallow in it. They really play it, and you can see it in the media, the glorification of narcissism. People will do anything to achieve fame. They'll confess to crimes they didn't even commit to get on television.

#3: Willingness to endure transitory anguish until the difficulty is transcended.

Spiritual work is sometimes difficult. To face one's inner feelings, sometimes you'll experience a state of disappointment at what you discover, like playing the victim. You look at what you're holding onto, and then you realize, to your dismay, that you're milking it and that you're really wallowing in victimhood. So, that transitory disappointment that you go through when you admit the truth of something to yourself is a temporary passing discomfort. You can see how selfish you are in a relationship. You can see how self-interested you are. You can see how indifferent you are. You can see how unloving you are in some areas. It becomes somewhat painful, the pathway of inner searching. That's why some people, like 12-Step groups, take a fearless moral inventory. It's often recommended that you have somebody to discuss it with so that you don't get hooked in some negative viewpoint and can't get out of it.

The Christian saints say how they went from elated states to states of despair: *"Oh my beloved, how could you have deserted me?"* Don't worry about the states of great anguish. Just surrender the anguish itself to God and constantly surrender all of it. Don't resist the anguish if it comes up, because if you're serious, it very likely will come up again.

I never knew anybody who just went into a state of happiness and stayed there all the way to enlightenment. Jesus Christ sweated blood in the Garden of Gethsemane. There's anguish along the way, but that experientially is what goes on and you say, "This too I'm willing to go through, oh Lord, whatever this anguish may mean or whatever it signifies."

Everybody along the spiritual pathway can benefit from having a mentor who, at times, can reflect back things that would be far more difficult to handle on your own.

#4: Constancy and watchfulness.

Mindfulness is being watchful and witnessing the phenomena going on in the mind. Many people are completely oblivious to their own mode and style of thinking and behaving. People can be shocked and offended all over the place by others, and they're not even aware they're being the same way: completely out of place, inappropriate, undiplomatic, not thinking of the sensitivities of others. With mindfulness, you become aware of your shortcomings, you honestly admit them, and then you ask God for help to overcome them.

The first thing is to become self-aware. Then, having become more self-aware, you're now more motivated to try to grow. Let's say you discover that you're really being quite selfish in every single interaction, so now you ask God to help you overcome this selfishness. When you ask God for help, you're opening a doorway of energy that wasn't there before. If you just ignore it, nothing much happens, but if you say, "Dear God, I am unable to overcome this self-interest and it seems to color everything I do. There must certainly be some great motivation that I could align with than just satisfying the personal ego." First of all, the personal ego is temporary, and when you leave the body, hopefully there's going to be something that's going to carry you further than the pits of the ego.

#5: Moving from self-interest as a participant/experiencer to that of the witness/observer.

If you are seriously interested in enlightenment, first you identify with the mind and think, *I am that.* You see yourself as the doer of all actions, and then you think, *Well, what is it that knows that?"* You realize it's because you're witnessing and observing it, so then you move and you see that you move to identify the witness/observer, and then from there, you move to the experiencer, which is a far more advanced and more refined thing to transcend, to stop identifying as the experiencer. However, it is relatively easy to see that that which you are as the witness and the observer, and then on an even more advanced level, you're the witness, the observer, and also the experiencer.

What you need to realize is those things are autonomous. There's no *you* that is witnessing. There's no *you* that is experiencing. There's no *you* that is observing. These are automatically happening of their own accord as a consequence of the nature of consciousness itself. It's *consciousness* that has all these capacities, not a personal *you*. We're talking about how to transcend identification with the ego, the pronoun of a personal self as a primary source of volition.

The ego wants to take credit for that which is actually spontaneous and automatic. It'd be like the ego always taking credit for the weather. "Well, I certainly did a nice job of today," it says. The sun is shining without you. But if it could get away with it, the ego would take credit for the sun shining.

#6: Willingness to relinquish judgmentalism and opinion about what is observed.

This is probably the hardest stage, because you see, our society itself is intrinsically narcissistic. The right to free speech and all that kind of thing—it's like everybody feels obligated to get out there and tell you how they feel about things. In reality, who cares what you feel about it? Nobody really gives a whit what you think or feel about it! I'll tell you why: Because they care about what they think or feel about it. They don't really care what you think about it. In fact, the only thing you do is add grist to their mill, so they can tell you how they think and feel about how you think and feel.

The idea is that by being truthful and integrous, you can't win. You have to manipulate it. We were saying the consciousness level of America has dropped. That's one of the reasons, the political dishonesty and the dominance of the media, which displays it all, and the seduction of all of that. That plus relativism, which allows it all to happen and have its blessing. If truth is no different than falsehood, then you can lie your head off and not feel guilty about it. You can say there is no such thing as absolute reality and no such thing as truth, and that everything is relative. Then you can avoid all kinds of guilt and you can be narcissistic for all your life without any responsibility. Some people project their own narcissism onto everything.

There are, however, many motivations that have nothing to do with narcissism. There are motivations having to do with merely being that which you are. Let's say you run marathons, and you enjoy them and you have the capacity to do them. Not everybody has the ability to do that. Another person could create music because it's the fulfillment of a potential. There are many motivations other than personal gain. There is fulfilling one's destiny. So there is a pleasure in being all that you can be to the greatest extent you can be, and that's a spiritual satisfaction of potentiality becoming an actuality, a fulfillment of a promise.

The human being is created with the capacity for the evolution of consciousness and the development of spiritual awareness, so the fulfillment of that potentiality then is the acknowledgment of a divine gift of the potentiality of life itself, and there is a gratification that comes from a knowingness of having fulfilled one's destiny. But I understand also what the critic says about it, that altruism and humanitarianism can also be accompanied by egocentricity. "Oh, look what a great donor I am. I've given my millions to the poor." Yes, and that does also happen. The two things can coincide. You can on the one hand be the integrous fulfillment of your potential and then the ego can also chime in and try to play off of it, and of course, that's so-called spiritual pride. People will become holier than thou. People become proud of their humility. "Look how humble I am!"

#7: Identifying with the field rather than with the content of the field.

This has to do with identifying with context—seeing that within the phenomena perceived to be occurring, you are not the content, you are the field. What is the infinite field of your ultimate reality? And that is consciousness itself. You're not the content of consciousness, you *are* consciousness. Without consciousness, you would not even be aware that you exist.

Did you know that below 200 people and animals do not really realize they exist? They are, but they do not comprehend that they are. A rabbit is, but it doesn't comprehend that it is. It's only over level 200 that you comprehend that you are.

#8: Accepting that enlightenment is one's destiny, understanding it is a condition that ensues as a consequence of decision, intention, and devotional dedication consequent to both karma and divine grace.

To avoid the spiritual ego, you stop seeing life as something to be accomplished, won, or succeeded at. You become that way because you're attracted to being that way, and not because you're driven by a goal. You become more loving when you let go of the limitations, the things that block it. A person doesn't just say, "I think I'm going to become more loving." You try to remove the obstacles to love—judgmentalism and various attachments and aversions.

People who are interested in spiritual work are really responding to an inner knowingness that, karmically, they are destined to reach higher levels of awareness. When I look at a lecture class, I'll ask, "What percentage of this class is destined for enlightenment?" They all are. Why? Who else would be in the class except people who are destined for enlightenment and how to reach enlightenment? Who would be in a class on golfing unless they're planning to go out on the green and golf? It's because there's an inner knowingness that you're attracted to, and that knowingness doesn't care what's involved. It just keeps pulling you like a current in that direction.

#9: Avoiding glamorizing or aggrandizing the endeavor or its destination and relying instead on devotion for its own sake.

This is about appreciating beauty for its own sake, not because by appreciating beauty, you're going to become something better or more accomplished. It's seeing the intrinsic value of a thing, and prizing it and valuing it because of its inner perfection. This is easier and easier as you go on, because you let go of blocks to it. You see the perfection and beauty of all things, and through revelation, the absolute perfection and the essence of divinity in all that exists shines forth with a stunning radiance. It's so stunning, it leaves the mind silent.

DIVINE LOVE AND PERSONAL LOVE

Personal love is looking for a gain, a gain of acquisition. It's solar plexus to solar plexus. With personal love, people are aligned by infatuation and craving: "I must have you or I will die." It's gratification, satisfaction, ownership, et cetera. Divine love is of the heart, and it's not personal. Divine love is a way of being in the world. Members of spiritual communities develop this love for each other. Men in the armed service develop a profound lifetime love for each other—a commitment to each other that transcends all gain. If you see a shipmate from 40 years ago, what happens is you break out in tears. This happened to me. Suddenly, the phone rang one day, and a voice at the other end was familiar, and instantly, I broke into tears. I said, "My God." Then I apologized for crying. He said, "Well, I've been contacting the remaining guys from the ship who are still alive. There's only five or six left. Each one, when I contacted them, every one of them cried like that. Don't feel embarrassed by it." That is a profound bond of love. Divine love is like a bonding. There's no gain involved. There's no gain in bonding. An old friend is an old friend, and the joy is simply in their presence.

Personal love is always looking for the seeking of a fulfillment of an instinctual drive. The craving for a need is coming out of the instinctual realm; that cravingness, desiringness, and feeling incomplete without something is an attachment and a trap.

LETTING GO OF THE DESIRE OF THINKINGNESS

The child is easily distracted by the phenomena in the world. It drives their parents crazy, because they are so distractible. You take them with you into the supermarket, and instantly they're lost between the aisles. They're checking out the merchandise on the shelves. No one transcends their distractibility, and we see that the child's distractibility is what gives the mind its attraction.

The adult is thinking all the time, because of the juice they're getting out of thinkingness. The way to stop thinkingness is to look at what you are getting out of that thinkingness. You energize the experiencer, for one thing.

When you look at what you're extracting out of thinkingness, you can let go of the desire of thinkingness and thinkingness will stop. Nothing there. And then you see that there's no one in the auditorium. The auditorium is empty and the infinite field is silent. The infinite field is silent when you stop wanting to attract thoughts; when you stop extracting any gain from them, they stop. The reason you think is because you want to think. You might say, "No, I don't want to think. I want my mind to be silent. I want to meditate." Well, that means that the gain, the desire is hidden from you, and you have to be more honest with yourself. You enjoy the entertainment. You enjoy the feeling that thinkingness gives you—a sense of existing and being alive, and that you are.

It's observing the illusion that you are a separate individual being having these unique thoughts. It's propping up the sense of an independent personal self. The child is dealing with perception, the witnessing of the visual phenomena. You might say a mystic would not be aware of the details, but they are witnessing the beauty of God's creation in this form, in the form of the clouds, the sky, the rain. Everything testifies to the presence of God as the source, an ongoing source of all of creation.

The divinity is then present in all things, not more in this than in that.

Chapter 9

ENLIGHTENED HEALERS

The further one progresses along the path of enlightenment, the more one becomes acutely aware of the profound relationship between mind and body. On the path of the ego, where the mind and body appear to be separate, the process of healing is treated with pills or delegated to doctors to fix the body; whereas on the path of enlightenment, one sees the mind and body as an integrated whole and understands that the mind, and even the soul, can play a profound role in healing a variety of conditions, from colds and allergies to depression and other forms of mental illness.

In this chapter, Dr. Hawkins will expand upon this profound understanding of what it means to be an enlightened healer.

So we've come up with this mathematical model in which the relative power of energy fields is calibrated so that you see that apathy, which is calibrated at 50, has only half the power of fear, which is calibrated at 100. Fear, on the other hand, has only half the power or energy of courage, which is calibrated at 200. Not only do these energy fields have different relative power to each other, but we see that the energy fields go in a certain direction. All the energy fields under courage are directed in a negative anti-life that which is oriented toward destruction. The energy fields below courage then tend to be anti-life in their effect.

At the level of courage, the needle swings to the midline, and as we go beyond the energy field of 200 up to neutral, willingness, acceptance, and love. These energy fields now go to the right, indicating that they nurture and support life, that they are energy giving, life giving, and they increase aliveness. As we go up the scale we go into energy fields of increasing aliveness, that which support life and the truth. As we get to the bottom of the field, we get to that which does not support life, which is anti-life, which does not represent the truth. Death is calibrated at zero.

At about 600, we leave the field of duality. We leave the field of illusion. We leave the identification with the small self, which is the ego in common parlance, and we move on into fields of enlightenment, so that the great enlightened beings, the great spiritual masters, the avatars, their energy fields begin in the 700s, and go on up into infinity.

The truth really indicates that which is supportive: supportive of life, supportive of aliveness. So when we're talking about health, we're talking about aliveness. What we're talking about is the expression of an energy field. The body expresses that which the mind holds. We're only subject to what we hold in mind. And therefore, the greater the negativity that is being held in mind, the greater the negative energy field effect on the body's physical health. The greater the positive energy being held in mind and consciousness, the more powerfully positive will be the energy field of life.

This gives us a tool now, a way of approaching things: does this support life, or does it not support life? We can substitute the word *health*, because health is nothing but the expression of life; we have energy fields that support illness, and we have energy fields that support life. Each of these energy fields reflects themselves in an emotion, so that which is anti-life, as you would expect, has negative emotions. These negative emotions include self-hatred, hopelessness, despair, regret, depression, worry, anxiety, cravingness, resentment, hatred, and arrogance. Negative emotions then accompany ill health. We see the process going on, in consciousness coming out of these emotional states: destruction, loss of energy, loss of spirit, deflation, entrapment, overexpansion, overinflation, loss of power.

We see the kind of world a person experiences out of these negative mental states. This is a world of sin and suffering, hopelessness, sadness, fear, frustration, and competition. It's a world of status. We see the negative conceptualizations of God that come out of a lower energy field. God is the ultimate enemy of man— the one who hates him, the destroyer, the one who throws him into hell forever. Or there's the God who ignores man. There's the God who's dead, who's punitive, who's retaliatory. We can then see how the negative view of the world and of God all correlate with ill health.

• • •

Illness is physical, mental, and spiritual. You can be spiritually ill and be physically well. Or you can be physically ill and spiritually well. Physical, mental, and spiritual—everything has a different dimension.

THE BENEFITS OF ILLNESS

It may be not necessarily a physical benefit, but there is a philosophic benefit to when you realize what you couldn't have lived with before is trivial and you *can* indeed live with it. You realize that you are far more than just your physical dimension. The physical dimension can be quite limited, and you can still be in a state of great happiness and spiritual grace in spite of it.

You can look at it in these ways, philosophically and spiritually, intellectually, and physically, and ask yourself, *What am I getting so nervous about? Or what is distressing me? What is it that I'm resisting?*

It could be that a person who is resisting is really experiencing out grief. They're *suppressing* the grief instead of just giving into it and weeping for a day or two, and then letting it all go. Don't forget everything that happens has a karmic antecedent. The grief you feel for a loss in this lifetime brings up all the grief of all the losses over all the lifetimes. People say, "Why am I so upset over this little thing?" Well, it isn't just this little thing. You've got a whole stack of suppressed feelings for many lifetimes, in which you didn't experience it out. There are resentments and angers and self-pities and God knows what else. So you could take advantage of it. When something comes up in this lifetime, feel it all the way until it finally runs out. If you're angry, you're not angry enough. Lay on the floor and pound your fist and scream and screech and squeal until all the angriness is gone, and do the same with the grief. And that way your vulnerability is lowered. If people are angry, I tell them the trouble is you're not angry enough. Go in the other room and scream and jump and shriek and clench your fists and pound the wall until you've got it all out.

People suppress those feelings; they don't like them. We're trained in a social way to repress them and not express them. And if you're a guy, you're not supposed to have grief or cry or anything like that. Let it go. Jump up and down and curse. Just go crazy with it. Finally, you can see it's ridiculous and it makes you laugh.

• • •

We have to look at the relationship between mind and body, because that is of great importance in the field of health, and it is one that is not really clearly understood. There is a certain principle, and it's demonstrated clinically, that we are only subject to what we hold in mind. Now, this is a principle of healing and a principle of health, two different sides of the same coin. Illness being one side of the coin, health the other. We're subject to what we're holding in mind. We see the illness then is coming out of a program, a belief system. The program went in and we are now subject to that for the rest of our life, with no memory of where that came from.

Because of childhood amnesia, many people can't remember what happened before the age of five. And some people even, at a much later age, they have no memory of anything from their entire childhood, or very few memories. Even for people with good memories of their childhood, there are vast areas of vacant forgottenness. And in those areas of vacant forgottenness are the many programs which are now expressing later on in various forms of ill health. You might hear things like, "Heart disease runs in our family," or "Allergies run in our family," et cetera. These thoughts then become a program and it goes into the mind and we see that it's the same as though the person was hypnotized. Until that program has made been conscious and canceled, it remains operative within the unconscious.

Now, why does the mind have such power over the body? Perhaps we can look at the physics of it a little bit. The physics would make it very easily understandable. We said in our calibrated system here that death is zero and guilt is 30. We can get the energy field of anything in the world. And so we calibrate the energy field of the body itself, and we find that the physical body is not a reversed state like this. The body is not a negative state, but the energy field of the body is about 100. In other words, its power, its energy field is about 100.

The energy field of mind begins around 400. It runs between 400 and 500. Those are the energy fields of the intellect, reason, logic, and what the mind believes. And therefore, if we hold a thought in the mind that says, *Seeds give me diverticulitis*, then the body, which only has an energy field of 100 is overpowered by the power of the pattern of that belief.

All thoughts have a form. And so the form, which is there in the collective unconscious, the collective consciousness, social consciousness, whatever you want to call it, is there in great detail. The pattern of that and the coming about of how the mechanics of that would happen is already there. If we buy into that thought, if we go into agreement with it, it's like we bring it into our own unconscious and that then expresses itself within the body. The body will do what the mind believes. The healing of the body then and the achievement of health, is achieved not by addressing the body directly, but by addressing the mind. Moving right into the fields of consciousness itself.

If the body is expressing that which is held in consciousness, then what we need to look at is what is being held in consciousness. Very often what's being held in consciousness, we are not aware of. In that case, we call it being unconscious of that. By looking at the body, we may have no recall of ever having had such a thought, but the body is telling us what must be. It's like an X-ray. The X-ray is telling us what must be held in mind for this to be presenting itself in the body. If the person, let's say develops clinical diabetes, and he says, "I don't remember anything in my family ever being said about that. Nobody in my family had diabetes. I don't see where it could have arisen in my mind." We know that somewhere in the unconscious is the belief in diabetes and all that goes with diabetes.

If we do research with an individual long enough and patiently enough, we will uncover where the program came from. But what it tells us is that the program is there, that the person thinks *I am subject to that*, and therefore, the healing has to be of the belief system. We have to heal where the origin of the illness starts. And so health comes out of mind. It comes out of positive mental attitudes. It comes out of a field of consciousness. It comes out of a level of consciousness, which expresses itself on the lower plane, the physical plane, as an expression of health coming out of these fields above neutral. Out of willingness, out of the willingness to be accepting, out of lovingness, out of inner joyfulness, and out of an inner state of peace.

That which is mental is in the 400s. Love is in the 500s, and of course spirit is 600 and above. So therefore, the intellect is not man's highest faculty, contrary to the age of reason and other learned works, or those intellectuals who hold that the thing that differentiates man from the animal is his intellect. The intellect is only in the 400s. There is something beyond mind, beyond logic, beyond reason, where it jumps and transcends into a whole different paradigm, a whole different way of being. It's necessary to know about that. It's necessary to know then that which heals. It's necessary to look at the contribution that is coming into an illness from these various levels.

We find that with an illness, if we don't understand the illness, then we will understand its reverse, which is health. These belief systems become self-reinforcing. They become self-fulfilling prophecies. We hold the belief, unwittingly, and it then manifests in our life. We look at that and we say, "See." And that justifies the belief system. By looking at our life, we can tell what beliefs we are holding. If we can't recall them, then we say they're unconscious. Therefore, our movement is upward in consciousness. We said health is the automatic expression of these higher energy fields. We see that gratitude is at 540, forgiveness is at 540, and healing is at 540. The willingness to be forgiving and grateful in itself automatically begins to heal.

• • •

We need to talk about the energy field of love and what it means. It's not sentimentality. What the world calls love is coming out of an energy field of dependency, control, sentimentalism, and emotionalism. An emotional, sentimental attachment in which there is control going back and forth, the satisfaction of desiringness on both sides, is called love. It's the Hollywood version. When you hear somebody say, "I used to love George, but I don't anymore," what they mean is that they never loved George. What that means is they had a sentimental attachment. Sort of a solar plexus, kind of a hanging onto, which the person then romanticized and glamorized within their life, and poured a lot of emotional energy into it. When that tie was broken, up came a lot of negative emotion.

The kind of love we're talking about is unconditional love. What is unconditional love? That's an inner decision that we make within ourselves. It's coming out of the intention and the decision to be a loving person. If I decide to love you, that is my inner decision. There is nothing you can do about that. Therefore, I am not the victim of what goes on in the world, because my decision to love creates a stable energy field of unconditionality. The other person's behavior may not please me, may not contribute to what I desire, but it doesn't change the lovingness. The mother, for instance, who visits her son who is a murderer in prison for 20 years, loves the beingness, the 'is-ness', that which the person really is. Of course, his behavior does not make her happy, but the love is unconditional, no matter what he does. So, the closest to it that we see in our world is the lovingness of the mother, which is unconditional.

I've often used the lovingness of 12-Step groups like Alcoholics Anonymous as an example of unconditional love. Unconditional love is not concerned with what you have. The people at the lower levels of consciousness are very concerned with havingness, and rate people back and forth on what they have. People are preoccupied with doingness. And people are rated and their status depends on what they do, and all the titles that go with their doingness. As you move toward the top, what people are concerned with is what you are, what you have become. Your is-ness, your beingness, that which you truly are. At that level, there is concern with a person's status, their value, the kind of person that you are, that which you have become. You have become that kind of person, and that is what is valued. The willingness then to become a forgiving person who nurtures all of life nonjudgmentally, automatically brings about within yourself, because of the very healing nature of that energy field, a condition of good health.

We're beginning to see the perfection of all things—how all things work out for the good. How can illness be held in that context? Illness becomes something that is coming up in order to be healed. We look at the illness then as a lesson. The illness is saying, "Look at me. Please heal what I stand for, what I symbolize. Please heal your guiltiness. Please heal your self-hatred. Please heal your limiting thought forms. Please move up to loving me so that I can be healed." The illness is a demand to grow spiritually. It's an incessant gadfly that tells us that something needs to be looked at. Something needs to be held in a different way. You see, because it is not the events of life, but how we hold them, that creates our reaction.

Events in and of themselves have no power to affect how we feel one way or another. It's what our position is about them. It's our *judgment* about them. It's how we decide to be with them. It's our attitude. It's our point of view. It's the context, the overall meaning, that gives the event the emotional power over us. We are the creator, then, of the meaning, and the impact that it has on us. Stress comes from that very thing. We give it power over our lives, coming from the position of victim, putting the source of happiness outside of our life, denying the power of our own mind. The healing comes about through the re-owning of the power, the realization that we and we alone create the meaning of any circumstance, event, place, position, thing, or person in our life. We are the ones who create the meaning. Our position, the way we hold it—that either becomes a source of healing or a source of illness. We are the ones who determine that.

We begin to see that the body is like a little marionette. It sort of happily goes about its way, coming out of these energy fields. It just sort of does what it does automatically, without much thinking. Being healthy means we pay less and less attention to the body and that which we do, which the world would call health-giving, is out of appreciation. It's an expression of how we are with that body. You see, we aren't giving away our power as source. Being healthy means you've re-owned your power as source. We're not giving away the source of health of the body to the world. The exercising we do is out of the joyfulness in experiencing the body. We don't say that swimming is what causes the body to be healthy. We come from the position that because we enjoy the body, we enjoy its activity such as swimming.

Those activities, which the world considers healthy, then are coming out of the expression of one's inner sense of aliveness. The joy is in allowing the body's expression in ways that the world considers healthy. It's not because they're causal; those expressions are the effect. The healthy enjoyment of the body, then, is the effect of the mental attitude. And therefore we come to a lovingness of the body. It's not a narcissistic self-glorification, or a muscle man picture in a magazine, but a pure lovingness and gratitude. We think, *Ah, body, you have served me well. I love you. I appreciate you. I value you.* If we put the source of our happiness on that which is outside of ourselves—our job, our possessions, our relationships—then we're merely setting ourselves up for the laws of our health.

What's going to come up, first of all, is fear of loss, even though that's not conscious. If the source of your happiness is your title, your address, the kind of car that you have, or even your physical body, you are now vulnerable. That vulnerability is in the unconscious, and it stores up a great deal of fear. Therefore, people's lives become endlessly about reinforcing and protecting themselves from the laws of those things upon which they have put their survival.

The healthy person realizes the true nature of who they really are—that they are something far beyond that. They realize that they are the ones that give those things value. Those things provide temporary enjoyment to them, but their survival doesn't depend on them. We said that when you move up into this energy field called acceptance, one has stopped giving one's power away to the world. One has begun to accept that I am the source of my happiness. If you put a person like that on a desert island and come back a year later, they'll have a coconut business going and they'll have found a new relationship, and they'll build a tree house in the tree, and they'll be teaching the children algebra. In other words, the capacity to recreate for themselves, the source of happiness comes from the realization that *I myself am the source of that happiness.* I myself am the source of health. It doesn't depend on epidemics, it doesn't depend on what is out there in the world. It doesn't depend on what I eat.

The healthy person realizes the true nature of who they really are—that they are something far beyond that.

When we really realize that, then we begin to transcend and no longer be at the effect of all these false belief systems. Consciousness itself requires something greater than itself, and that we call awareness. Awareness is what allows us to know what is going on in consciousness, reporting what is happening within mind, which in turn is reporting what is happening via the senses about the body. That which is essentially myself, then, is many levels removed from the physical body. And it's necessary for us to look at that and get that correctly in mind, because now we see that it's the mind that has power over the body. We see the physics of it, that the energy fields of the 400s just by their sheer power are greater than that of the physical body.

The physical body does what the mind tells it to do. And therefore, if the mind says, *I have this disease or that disease*, the body complies. When we look at this, we see the importance then of not buying into programs, all of which are really limitations of the truth. We see the importance of consciously canceling and saying something that is the truth. The truth is, "I am an infinite being, not subject to that."

Let's say we're told that eggs are full of cholesterol, and cholesterol will give you heart disease. If you buy into the thought form, that belief system, what happens is that the body agrees. You can experiment with this because I've done it. And at one time I had very high cholesterol. And I began to cancel the belief system. I kept saying, "I'm an infinite being. I'm not subject to that. I'm only subject to what I hold in mind. This does not apply to me. And I hereby cancel it and refuse it." If the mind can empower you with a negative belief system, it can reverse itself. Therefore, you begin telling yourself that they have no effect on you, that that's only a belief system.

When I go into agreement with a belief, I give it the power of the collective energy of that belief. When I refuse it, then I release myself from the collective energy of that belief system. One attitude then is to not buy into agreement with negative belief systems having to do with your health. This is very important when it comes to epidemics, the hysteria. The programming that comes in is aided and abetted by an emotional program. All of this contributing then is setting the stage. You have the mental belief system coming out of an energy field in the 400s, you have fear about it coming out of a negative 100s, and you have the guilt coming out of the minus 30s. You have the exact setup for that, because the mind will choose that which it is impressed with. It will use that as a form of expression. In the case of the cholesterol, the experiment I did with that, with my own self, was to cancel the thought every time it came up. And as time went by, the cholesterol level came down, and I could then eat three eggs for breakfast every single morning, with lots of cheese. I live on a high cholesterol diet, and yet my cholesterol is low, sometimes even below normal for my age.

The body will do exactly what the mind believes. And, of course, we have a credibility problem here. The person says, "Oh, how could just my belief in that make it happen within my life?" It's because of the nature of the unconscious. It creates the opportunity for that to happen. We certainly see that in accidents. If the person is accident prone, that's the form that it has taken in that person's mind. Unconsciously, they just managed to get their body into the right place at the right time to get hit by the fender of the car, slip down the stairs, or get hit in the head. Don't worry about how the mind will find a way. The mind will find a way. People will just slip into sort of a hypnotic trance and expose themselves to the correct opportunities to make that manifest within their life.

We know for instance, with the cold virus, there's many experiments where we take 100 subject volunteers, and expose them to a very heavy dose of cold virus. And we see that not everybody gets the cold virus. Only a certain percentage will always get it, only certain percent. In other words, if the power was in the virus rather than within consciousness, all 100 would get it, because that virus would be so potent. Actually, what happens is maybe only 65 percent will get it, a third don't believe in it. There is sufficient doubt within the mind. There's insufficient, unconscious guilt. It's not acceptable to the person to express it in that form. And so nothing is universal. We see the same thing with healings.

Every medical treatment has only a certain percentage of people who will respond. And what is the difference? It is because the others don't have sufficient unconscious guilt. It's not operative. This particular illness doesn't fit any particular thought form that they have bought into. Both sides of it, the sickness and the healing, are reflecting then the energy that we've put into a certain belief system. We see then that health is the willingness to let go of buying into negativity.

Why should a person buy into negativity anyway? Why is it some people are so programmable? We know people that go into hysteria every time they open a magazine. The latest illness sends them into a panic. And it has to do then with the amount of fear and the amount of guilt. The amount of fear is really coming out of the amount of unconscious guilt. It's as though the person knows what to be afraid of. It's as though they're only too aware that because they have so much of this, for them to even hear about it and become mentally programmed, is almost enough to make it happen in their life.

What does this tell us then about the steps toward optimal health? We see power in the willingness to adopt mental attitudes that are positive and constructive, and letting go of the negative ones. We see how buying into negative programming impacts the power of mind. Going into denial and blaming it on others is giving your power away. We see that these energy fields below courage are all levels in which the person has become a victim. What's happened is they've given their power away and put it on something outside of themselves. And these people in these lower levels have said to themselves unconsciously, the source of my happiness is outside of myself. They've put their survival on something outside of themselves.

As we move into the levels of truth above the levels of courage, and the energy fields are now going positive, we see that the person is re-owning their power. The person is saying, "I and I alone have the power to create happiness and opportunity in my life. It is coming from within me." And so these people then own that health is something that comes from within. They see they are not the victim of viruses, accidents, cholesterol, or uric acid levels. They're not the victim of those things.

When we re-own our own power, we say, "Hey, it's my mind that's been creating that. My mind believes that eating liver and kidneys is going to give you a high uric acid level, and that's going to give you an attack of gout. My mind is so powerful that if I believe that it will literally make it happen." That's a hard thing for many people to accept, that their mind has that much power.

• • •

The next thing the mind says is, "I don't want to give up the pleasure of eating." Sounds like you're going to come into a loss, right? You're not going to be able to enjoy a malted milk or hot fudge sundae or a hamburger smothered in onions? Quite the contrary. What happens to the enjoyment of eating once you do this is that appetite arises out of the eating itself. I'll sit down with no hunger and no appetite at all. But the minute I begin to eat, it creates appetite. And the pleasure of eating is more than it ever was. I enjoy food now more than I ever did, because it's not accompanied by guilt anymore. It's not accompanied by self-blame or anxiety. I don't worry if I'm eating too many calories or going to gain weight. Those worries are eliminated. So you're not going to give up the pleasure of eating at all. You'll find that when you eat, that you're enjoying the food considerably. You start enjoying the food the minute you take a bite. There's no loss of enjoyment. I don't believe in letting go of enjoyment and pleasure. On the contrary, I believe in increasing it.

You can have the enjoyment and the pleasure of eating, as well as the enjoyment and pleasure and pride in having a body that's more appropriate to your own aesthetic ambitions. It has nothing to do with your self-worth. It has nothing to do with the fact that you're self-indulgent. It has nothing to do with oral narcissistic needs or whatever the psychoanalytic theory might be—oral aggression, oral passivity—it's got nothing to do with that. It merely has to do with this simple, very primary type of conditioning, which has been favored in our society. You picked it up from your own social conditioning as a child. That's all. The body is experienced in mind, and the mind is experienced in consciousness. Where you're really experiencing that, what you've called hunger in the past, is in your consciousness. And where is that localized? You'll notice that it's only a belief system that hunger is experienced in the stomach. It's actually experienced everywhere. The thought that it is in the stomach is just a belief system from childhood. The body cannot experience anything. Hunger is experienced in a more diffused, generalized area.

Another technique in letting go of suffering of any kind, whether it's pain or illness or physical symptoms (in this case, what we've been calling hunger), is knowing that it is nothing but a physical symptom. As I said, it is being experienced in a diffused kind of way. It's being experienced everywhere. Because where do we experience all experience? Actually, it's being experienced in an everywhereness rather than a localized situation. The localization is coming from the strong belief systems. We have all these thoughts from childhood. As we let go resisting the energy of this sensation, it finally disappears.

• • •

It's generally thought that these negative feelings are the cause of weight problems. If you look into it, you'll see, this is really not so. You'll see that negative feelings are the *reaction* to the weight problem. Most of us have been down at the level of guilt. Guilt is an energy field of 30. It's very weak. If you try to handle your weight problem or any problem at all—alcohol, relationships, you name it—from the level of guilt, you can see how much energy you've got to work with. You've got like 30 bucks, as compared to love, which is 500 bucks. So, 30 bucks isn't going to buy you much progress in anything. Not only that, but the energy field is negative, meaning you're going to feel lousy about the whole thing. You're going to be full of self-hatred, and actually the process itself is destructive. People have actually committed suicide over their weight problems, their self-indulgence. Even if you don't handle it from guilt, you move up to hopelessness, which has an energy field of 50. This means my case is hopeless. I've tried all the diets. I've lost the energy to even address this problem anymore. I'm the victim of it, and I just surrender to it and give up. I am hopeless.

The next level above it is grief. This is the depression about the problem: the regret, feeling despondent and dispirited, or the fear of the problem and its consequences. These are all negative feelings, which include thoughts like *I'm going to die of a heart attack* or *This disease is going to kill me*. This field is full of worry, anxiety, and panic. And of course your self-esteem is deflated. People with a weight problem often socially withdraw. They compensate in other ways because they feel inadequate due to this energy field. They're not inadequate people at all; it's just that they're holding that about their situation, and then the negativity of it affects their emotions.

And we move up to the next field, which is anger. The person is angry about their weight problem, they resent it, they're full of grievances about it. At 150, they're probably going to be more effective utilizing anger—certainly instead of guilt or hopelessness. If you're angry enough about your weight problem, you can move up to pride, which is 175. There's a lot of power in pride, but you try to move through pride. It's not exactly a great place to hang out in, because of the inflation of the ego that happens there, so you hopefully move up to courage.

Now that you know some tools that are really going to work, you have the courage to try them out. Courage is at 200, which is a lot of power as compared to 30 or 50. Courage enables you to face, to cope, to handle, and what happens there is you become empowered. The truth of it is, you haven't known how to handle it up to now, otherwise you would have handled it. That's the truth of it. You use these releasing techniques, these letting-go techniques, and you become detached from the whole problem. If the weight stays, it stays, and if it doesn't stay, it doesn't make any difference. At this point, you say, it's not apathy, it's not hopelessness.

On the other hand, you're released from the weight problem, and therefore you're feeling good, and you move up to a willingness.

Willingness at 310 is a lot of energy. Compare it to guilt, compare it to grief. You see how much power you've got now. And here you're in agreement, you're aligned with this technique. Your intention is finally up. You're finally going to handle it, and you accept that it can be handled. You realize that you're an adequate person, and you start becoming confident. And there's a transformation now occurring because you realize the power to handle this is within you and you start moving up into lovingness. The desire to really love yourself. To love this body, now that you don't identify with it as *me*. This body is not me. You take off my left leg, I'm still me. You get that the me is me, and I'm not the body. So whether it weighs 200 pounds, or 85 pounds, that which I am is unassailable, and I must learn to love that body now. You begin to really value it, and see that it's just an enjoyable little puppet. The body goes about its way, and the less attention you pay to it, the better it really handles itself. It just does what it's doing automatically.

And if you get to love the body, your brain begins to release endorphins. When endorphins are released, a process goes on in consciousness called revelation. You begin to see things differently. What do you see differently? You see how wonderful your little body is. You begin to love it and get a kick out of it. When you're overweight, are you getting a kick out of your body? No. Every time you look at it, it throws you back into guilt again. At this level, you start getting a kick out of it. You start getting playful with it, sort of a joyfulness. A joyfulness and a happiness about the body. It bounces around, and you're just sort of dimly aware of it, because you're experiencing your existence from a position of allness. Once you become conscious about where experience is happening, you get that experience is happening everywhere. You begin to identify with everywhereness, instead of stomachness or bulgeness, all those localized things. That which I am is a conscious being. Consciousness is everywhere. I begin to experience my existence as being almost everywhere in space.

We start to come from the Heart about it then. Heart with a capital *H*. Heart not meaning the physical organ, Heart meaning that quality of valuing your existence. Coming from that greatness, coming from the bigness, coming from the joy of aliveness, and seeing the body as a contributor to that, as something that's enjoyable. It's something that you can have fun with, something you can play with, and something to have a good time with. It's really fun to sit down and watch this phenomena happen. It's really joyful. Within a day or two, it's all over. Within a couple of days, once you're released off this appetite hunger cycle, the rest of it is automatic. You don't have to do another thing.

It's different than being at the effect of, or run by the guilt. Now you have choice. Another trick that works is to put an envelope inside your refrigerator. In the envelope, place a picture of yourself as you as an adult, so that you remember you've got a choice of whose arm is going to be reaching into the refrigerator. Keep the kid out, because the kid is going to help himself to whatever he wants.

The whole thing becomes a very enjoyable experience, one in which you truly begin to love yourself. The basis of all these self-healing techniques that we talk about are merely ways of loving yourself, ways of really beginning to value yourself, and that which you really are in truth.

You'll see that the mind, the ego has played a trick on you. You think that you make a decision, and then the body does that. Actually, it's doing it by itself, it's on automatic. Once you've released it out of a negative pattern, the body will just handle itself very well. We know this with scientific experiments with young children. If you allow them to spontaneously select their diet, they will automatically select a balanced diet. So you begin to get a return of faith in nature. You allow the body now to sort of be itself. That which is natural within the body itself will automatically handle its nutritional needs.

Once we get off the social programming, then that which is automatically self-healing and healthy within the body takes over. It looks after itself, and it chooses what it needs to eat and what it wants to eat. And it does extremely well. My body eats lots of cho-lesterol, and it loves cheese and eggs, and my diet would make any dietitian faint. Any nutritionist I'm sure would faint when they see what I have for breakfast. And yet the cholesterol is normal, the blood sugar is normal, all the blood chemistries are normal. I have a faith, then you might say, in the God within nature itself, with the body being part of the beautiful nature of this planet.

• • •

One of the best ways to handle depression is to discuss it with other people. People will give you feedback. There's a trust in the general human energy. There is really a surprising willingness to help other human beings. I discovered that in New York City. For instance, if you're feeling down and you're standing outside of a building and there's a doorman, and you say to the doorman, "I don't know what's wrong with me, I'm really feeling down today," surprisingly, the doorman will usually say to you, "Yeah, I get those periods too and here's what I do about it . . ." There's a general helpfulness in mankind that you don't realize until you call upon it.

I think joining a therapeutic organization can also help. Peo-ple go to church, or group therapy, where there is some kind of group dynamic. The 12-Step groups have been one of the most profoundly powerful ways of overcoming a great variety of prob-lems, social isolation among others. There are great many ave-nues for help in today's world that really didn't exist when I was younger.

• • •

There's actually a physiologic change in the brain that occurs as a result of becoming spiritually oriented, spiritually committed, joining spiritual groups, practicing spiritual principles, just simply praying, genuflecting—all things that are symbolic of acknowl-edgment of the presence of God as divinity. They begin to trans-form you. You begin to experience and see the world differently.

A lot of people live in pride. Let's take spiritually oriented people: at 500 and over, the chances are probably 90 percent that you're relatively happy. You're so used to being happy that if you're not happy for a moment, you think you're unhappy. When you get a negative thought like that you ask God to remove it, "Dear God, please help me to get over this angry thought, and replace it with a pleasant thought."

I believe calling upon God is the most powerful and effective energy field that's available to you. And then because of divinity, you then have the courage to speak to another human being about the fact that you're feeling down, and you get a chance to talk about it. And when you talk about it, somehow the feeling diminishes. Any feeling that you have, if you talk about it, eventually you run it out. You can only feel so depressed about a certain number of things, and after you get through talking about it, you sort of work out that depression.

That's one of the reasons psychotherapy works, because you have a chance to share your concerns with another human being, and a psychotherapist has your well-being as his or her primary goal. It's useful.

ACTIVE AND PASSIVE SUICIDE

Passive suicide is not resisting the negative within you. Active suicide is seeking it. There's more of an emergency response. The active suicide is more like an emergency response of desperation. Passive suicide is more failing to take the necessary measures to survive. And of course, passive suicide is a guiltless way of doing it, whereas active suicide would make you feel guilty. There's a moral objection to active suicide. Passive suicide is a way of getting around the moral dilemma and being able to excuse it. That it's the world that did it, not you. People stop eating, and they stop taking whatever medications they need, and they don't do what's necessary to survive.

If you picture the source of happiness is something out there, well, what happens if you lose that something out there? The title, money, job, relationship? Again, you have to see that the source of happiness is really within you. Even if there was something outside of you, that was only the trigger. The source of happiness was still within you, and the accomplishment of something in the external world merely released it. What it released is the capacity to experience happiness that emanates from within. And all the external was, was a trigger.

In other words, money can't make you happy. If I say to somebody, "Here's a million dollars," and I hand them a briefcase full of money, the person feels instantly happy. But their life doesn't change. They're just sitting in the same chair, with the same bills. It's the thought—the thought that now they're suddenly going to be rich—that makes them very happy. What made them happy was this wild and crazy thought that money is going to make them happy.

It wasn't the money, after all; it was the thought of it. If you put the source of happiness in something outside of you, then you live in the fear of losing that whatever it is outside of you. If you see that the source of happiness is only within yourself, all the external did was release something that is internal to begin with. Nothing out there can make you happy. Nothing can make you happy in the world. Why? Because happiness radiates from within. All I could do is trigger that potentiality within you. If I tell you there's a lot of money in this case, and I'm putting it up in the closet, and if you need it, it'll always be here, you'll feel happy. You'll feel safe and secure. It doesn't have anything to do with whether there's real money in there or not. The *belief* that there's money in there is all you need.

There was a famous story from many years ago, Mama's Bank Account. A family was very worried during the Great Depression. Everybody was very poor, and sort of panicked. Mama said, "Well, don't worry about it because if we really needed the money for that, I'll get it from my bank account." Everybody would calm down. The son said, "If I lose my job, we're not going to be able to pay the rent." Mama went, "Never mind, I'll get it from my bank account." The family would lose this fear from *just the idea of it*, that Mama's bank account could solve their problems. And then after Mama finally died, they found out she never even had a bank account.

Underneath the depression, there is a fear or a combination of fears. And one way out of the depression is to look at all the fears that you're handling, and forget about the depression and just handle the fears. And if you handle the fears and look at the fears and resolve them, the depression will disappear. So clinically, depression is always based on a fear: a fear that you're not good enough, that you will not accomplish, a fear of the future, a fear of God's punishment, a fear of self-approval. If you handle the fears, the depression will disappear.

• • •

Health then comes out of a positive mental attitude. That's the thing we've heard many times, haven't we? In fact, many people are annoyed by this idea, because that infers if I have a sickness, I don't have a positive mental attitude. Let's look at mental attitude then. Let's look at what is meant by that and the part that plays in health, and freedom of sickness and suffering.

We said the one thing that goes on in the unhealthy person is this unconscious guilt. The cure for that is the willingness to be forgiving, to actually take courses in forgiveness if that is necessary, such as *A Course in Miracles*, which is specifically designed to let go of that tendency of the mind, to criticize, to attack, and to judge. The willingness then is to let go of judgmentalism. Now the mechanism is unconscious. The person may not see the connection between the fact that their mind is critical, judgmental. If your mind is critical and judgmental of others, of course, it is critical and judgmental of yourself.

The creation of the unconscious guilt then goes up a certain energy which expresses itself through the autonomic nervous system, and the acupuncture energy system. That is the cure of that. The contribution from mind, the belief system, we said is the power of refusal to deny it. The willingness to own back your power now, that it is the mind and the mind itself that is the cause of the illness. The willingness to give up the position of victim. The willingness to re-own one's own power is part and parcel of the third thing that's necessary for health, and that is one's overall spiritual growth and development. It is the overall moving out of these negative energy patterns, the willingness to face truths within ourselves, and the moving into a positive energy field.

This can be done rather rapidly. How so? Because willingness, you see, is the key. Through the willingness to look at it, the willingness to say, "Well, I don't really believe this, but it is said that my mind has the power to create an illness within my body. So I'm willing to look at that, because I have an open mind. I have an open mind, and I'm willing to agree my intention aligns then, and I begin to move into accepting that which I discover. I begin to find that moving into a lovingness has a curative and healing power." And how do we do that? We do that with our willingness to forgive, and if we do that we can quickly move ourselves into the willingness to be compassionate.

What does compassion mean? Compassion means the willingness to see the innocence within all things. That coincides with the willingness to forgive. Out of compassion comes the power, the capacity, coming out of our intention, to really see into the hearts of others. And when we see into the hearts of others, what we discover is the innocence of the child within each and every one of us. Because it is intrinsic to the nature of consciousness itself, that intrinsic innocence, which never dies, no matter how long we live. The innocence of the child is what brought the mistake, which brought the negative program in the first place.

It's being aware that that intrinsic innocence of the child is ever with us. It's the innocence of the child that sits there in front of the television set, and buys the negative programming, out of its naivete, out of its lack of discernment. The innocence of the child has no warning within it. Nothing within the innocence of the child thinks, *This is a world that is out there to program you with as much negativity as you're willing to buy.* In fact, it gets well paid to do that, because advertising is usually based on playing off of these negative energy fields—all of our fears, all of our desires, all of our pridefulness. The willingness then is to be aware that within us is our innocence, and understand that the innocence needs to be protected.

We come into what's called self-care. Self-care, the capacity to love oneself now, means taking responsibility to protect ourselves from that innocence, and the willingness to undo the mistakes that the mind picked up as a result of its innocence. We can handle now looking at ourselves and healing that which we find within us, if we're coming from the compassion of the awareness of the intrinsic innocence of our consciousness. We see that it was innocence that God programmed. Now we take responsibility for that and we say, "Well, in my innocence, I bought all that. In my innocence, I didn't know any better. In my innocence, I thought that the right thing to do was to be judgmental, to condemn people, to judge them as right and wrong. Now, I see that that has made me sick, and so I'm going to let it go."

This capacity then to be forgiving is within us. The capacity for compassion, out of it comes a general attitude, a way in which we look at ourselves. From our bigness, from our greatness, we look at our humanness through forgiving eyes, and we begin to forgive ourselves for all the things that were limitations and denials of the truth.

The body is reflecting what the mind believes, and the mind is reflecting our spiritual position. Spirit has the greatest power of all. And therefore, our spiritual position literally determines whether we will have a healthy physical body or not. Once we're willing to accept the power of mind, now we have to be attentive, and we have to persevere, and we can't let it get away with expressing negativity without stopping it. We get to develop an ear for negativity and begin to recognize it for what it is. We let go of false humility, and we start questioning such remarks like, *I'm not very bright* or *My handwriting is poor* or *I gained so much weight*.

The minute we hear ourselves saying these limiting, self-defeating, self-attacking thoughts, they have to be stopped and canceled. The handwriting is poor, because there's a belief system that I have poor handwriting, and not vice versa. What we're doing then, is reversing the whole programming of the mind as far as cause and effect. We're coming back to a principle that you can demonstrate through your own experience, that the physical is the expression of the mental, and not vice versa. It isn't that we came to the conclusion that our handwriting is poor because our handwriting is poor. The handwriting is poor because the cause was in mind, the belief system, perhaps a remark picked up in childhood. Somebody says your handwriting is poor, from that point on that program now becomes operative.

Chapter 10

ENLIGHTENMENT

In this final chapter in The Wisdom of Dr. David R. Hawkins, *Dr. Hawkins expands his view from one of individual enlightenment to enlightenment on a national and global level. And as you'll learn in the sections that follow, enlightenment on any level of life experience is achieved by applying the same spiritual principles.*

The challenge for each of us is to become an enlightened leader ourselves, so we can inspire a generation of enlightened leaders, who can help to raise the calibration level of our country, and ultimately our world.

Dr. Hawkins begins this section by discussing the ever-divided political climate, and concludes on a spirit of unity with a prayer to send you happily and courageously further down the path to enlightenment.

In recent years, the political dialogue has calibrated at consciousness level 200. In my generation, the political dialogue calibrated at about 280 or 290, so it's of a lower nature now. It's just on the edge of 200, neither good nor bad, but at the same time, neither one.

It's because of the influence of the media, which we just discussed in the previous chapter. People are not interested in what you are in reality. They're interested in what kind of an image is projected of you. The projected image is what they are hoping will sway the populace. And as I say, it's done by popularity, not by capability. It's like being the most popular surgeon on the staff. It doesn't mean you're the best one. When I get operated on for a brain tumor, I'm not interested in a popularity contest, I'm interested in expertise.

Our society is not looking at expertise; they're looking at popularity. They figure popularity is what gets the votes, so the aim of the political dialogue then is being very conscious of the media and then trying to play the media and play to people's prejudices and belief systems rather than lead them. Some people think this is a great emergence forward, but it is not. It's just a play on popularity. We have sexism and racism, and then, of course, we have ageism. All these -isms are battling for each other. As we say, the minute you add -ism to the end of a thing, it drops below 200. The actual impact of the dialogue is below 200. In the media, we see people trying to suppress certain things and amplify other things. It's sort of the usual manipulation.

The desire for political office is ravenous, and once people are bitten by it, it seems like they will do or say anything to get into that office. As I say, the minute you get elected, 50 percent of the people hate you because they all voted against you. Why the office is so popular is hard to say . . . narcissism, I guess.

I would view the office as being one of responsibility, that you're elected because of the recognition of your capability to be the best leader at the time. And of course, I, having lived through a different generation, I remember the start of World War II. Winston Churchill was drafted to be who he was because of his capability, not his popularity. After winning the war, in the next election, after saving their lives, the populace did not vote him in. That was the thanks he got, the thanks he got for engineering the winning of the war and holding the British people together. With consciousness level 500, they didn't even re-elect him! That was a real kick in the head, wasn't it? You sacrifice everything for your country to save your country, and they don't even re-elect you, which is what I think about politics.

Integrity is upfront; character and integrity plus capability. You would want somebody with great experience and great integrity and a good sense of reality, who understands politics and who's been in it long enough. You'd just be looking for positive characteristics. Now, none of those characteristics have anything to do with race or gender. Gender doesn't make you a better politician, neither does race or color or age or any of those things, any more than it would make you a better physician. I don't care what color a brain surgeon is. I want the best brain surgeon around.

• • •

The political form of democracy doesn't last more than a couple of hundred years. And sometimes it only survives because it's restricted or put in other directions. Democracy is how old in our country? And it still seems to be operating quite well. But the more ignorant people, the more selfish people, the people who have lower levels of consciousness, are going to vote based on personal gain. They are not voting for the good of the community, the good of the populace, out of good will, or health, or public relations, but out of selfishness.

Calibration levels below 200 are all narcissistic. It's all me, me, me, what can *I* get? The higher the level of it, the greater the percentage of the population is below 200, the greater the danger to the survival of democracy. At this point, they neglect their duties to society, to their fellow Americans. They make decisions based on certain intrinsic values.

So when we talk about raising consciousness, it sounds sort of purposeful, like we're going to do this and then the consciousness is going to raise. But what you do is you reaffirm the value of that which is integrous. You reaffirm it by constant respect.

WAR AND PEACE

People think war and peace are opposites. They're not opposites at all. People think if nobody's getting shot, you have peace. You don't have peace. Because that which lives off war is very alive. In fact, war has peace demonstrations.

Peace is the natural state when truth prevails. It's the field. In the field itself, the natural state is peace. When truth prevails, you automatically have peace. War has nothing to do with violence. It has to do with the automatic condition when falsehood prevails. The opposite of war is not peace. Therefore, the basis of war, if it's falsehood, would be ignorance, the inability to tell truth from falsehood.

Peace is the natural state when truth prevails.

The stunning thing about *Power vs. Force*—I can say that because there's no me to feel egotistical about it, I was simply the witness to the writing of *Power vs. Force*—was it discerned for the first time in all of human history how to tell the truth from falsehood. The karma of mankind changed with that book. Until that point, nobody, nowhere in time could tell the difference between truth and falsehood, except an advanced mystic, and they stayed in safe places. They didn't get on the front lines.

The basis of war then is ignorance. When you watch the history of Nazi Germany on the History Channel, how the Hitler Youth grew up, it breaks your heart because they thought they were going to Boy Scout camp. They had fires and they held hands and they did brave things for the fatherland. You can see the innocence. The human mind is incapable of telling truth from falsehood because it's only hardware. And what society puts in is software. The hardware is unchanged. *A Course in Miracles* says innocence is untarnished no matter what. The hardware is not affected by the software. Society puts in the software.

You can take these innocent children. In the last century, 100 million people have died because of that innocence, 100 million. And Jesus Christ said, "There's only one problem: ignorance. Forgive them. They know not what they do." Ignorance. Buddha said, "Only one sin, ignorance."

THE 7 STEPS TO BENEFIT THE WORLD

#1: Form an Advisory Council

Well, this isn't going to please everyone, but any kind of academic study or clinical study comes out with recommendations at the end, based on these findings. As I have recommended, before you invest money in research it is very important to calibrate the level of integrity of the research design, the researcher, the intention of the study. We did a study in international politics, the levels of various governments, types of government, political leaders going all the way back in history. We ended up with what we thought was maybe a basic structure for a science of diplomacy based not on perception and the media image, but on the reality. Studying our own society from a political viewpoint and others, and looking at the history of war, and analyzing the details of various wars, you see, we arrived at some suggestions.

The level of knowledge of the affairs about which they legislate among politicians is extremely low. For instance, they pass laws on medicine and all kinds of aspects of society, international commerce, et cetera, and yet their knowledge of these things is abysmal.

The catastrophes of society and civilization have been made over and over again. If we calibrate the various forms of government, we find that democracy is near the top, but not the actual top. Interestingly, we find that a government based on an advisory council, or a so-called oligarchy, calibrates even higher. An advance of five degrees or five points is quite significant. If we look at political systems, we just calibrate them abstractly. We see that oligarchy at 415 is the highest of all these areas. Democracy is at 410, which is quite high. Iroquois Nation is about 400, coalition 345, socialism 300, monarchy 200, et cetera. It goes down from there.

Oligarchy is a very ancient system. It's not familiar to Americans. The survival of most tribal society is based on the wisdom and sagacity of the tribal elders, who are revered. The chief is not the same as the oligarchic council of the elders. What our country seems to lack is a council of elders. We have a cabinet. All the political power positions are political appointees. What's important is which party you belong to and who your friend is and who are you obligated to. In essence, who do you have to pay off? Because of my own particular alignment toward integrity and truth, and what is beneficial to society and the world, without any particular positionality, my belief is that we need a council of the elders. Now, the equivalent of a council of the elders is an advisory council.

In the old days, a true oligarchy, the council of the elders, has the power. Because of the nature of our government, this really couldn't be operationally done. Our constitution is not set up for that. However, something beyond the cabinet level is needed. This has to be made up of statesmen and not politicians. A statesman calibrates much higher than a politician, because the politician has an agenda. A statesman, Churchill, held together the British people during World War II. That's a spiritual energy, you see.

An advisory council is composed of people who have nothing more to gain. They've got it made. They don't need anything. So what do you do when you've got it all? You offer yourself to be of service. Take people who've been extremely successful in business: They don't need any more money, titles, or power. But they do have wisdom. How do you build the biggest giant corporation in the world? How do you make General Motors run?

You take the wisdom of these people who have nothing personally to gain, which they share with each other about the country's problems, and then they're available as consultants to the politicians. They're not going to tell you what to do, but they will see that if you make this move, you're forgetting about this other consequence. A real statesman would point out, "I would make that move, but I would do it slow so that you don't create the opposition. You're going to create a counter wave. You're going to defeat yourself. You're going to get the propositions through the first vote. But then the repercussion is going to hit, and they're going to wipe you out again."

The advisory council is there to guide in policy and decision-making because they can contextualize it, tell you what's the upside, the downside.

#2: Learn how to diagnose malignant messianic narcissism, and thereby identify and counter dangerous leaders before they threaten the world.

This is crucial. This is a matter of public education. As you get more advanced, then the capacity to recognize and identify this psychopathology, parading as some politician, grows. If people are attuned and aware of this, they begin to recognize it early in the game, not after the narcissists have established the Gestapo or the OGPU, not after they've killed off all the best generals, not after they've exterminated all the intellectuals, and not after they've transported all the Jews out of Germany, not after they've sacrificed all kinds of things in their society. Then, belatedly, they might say, "Oh boy, did we ever make a mistake?" The death of 10 million. It takes the death of 10 million people before people begin to wonder, "Gee, I wonder if we made the right decision."

That's one thing that an advisory council does, is make people aware in the diplomatic world of what it is you're dealing with. You hear silly propositions like, "If we're sweet and nice to them, they'll love us." You know that's ridiculous. If you calibrate that right now, you'll get no. The malignant kind of pseudo masculinity hates the feminine. You're talking from the feminine to a consciousness that *hates* the feminine. You calibrate the position of women and children in those repressive, totalitarian cultures, and they're about the level of dogs. They're not allowed to own anything, go out in public, go anywhere, be anything. To survive then, there has to be a means to recognize and diagnose malignant messianic narcissism before it's out of hand, because once they've killed off all the intellectuals, and all the people who are capable of recognizing it, it's too late.

The cost of not being able to recognize and diagnose malignant messianic narcissism cost 100 million lives in the last century. In my lifetime, 100 million people went to their deaths for this one single ignorance. And it's so easy to diagnose.

#3: Identify dangerously fallacious ideologic trends before they become epidemics.

Fallacy masquerades as truth, and the naive mind, and especially the evil mind, is unable to discern truth from falsehood. That which can be sold as plausible is sold as chic, superior, and elite. And it's brought down the calibration level of the integrity of academia. And now you see academics saying things that are so outrageous that even a grade school child wouldn't believe it, and they're taking it seriously.

We have a different syndrome, you see, and that is the distortion of truth to subserve egoistic ends. In my books, we've traced recent philosophies, calibrated all the most prominent philosophers who promulgate the various versions of relativism, and what you end up with is the distorted hermeneutics of relativistic epistemology. In layman's terms, that means how to distort truth in such a way that you're like Alice in Wonderland and you say, "Well, the thing means what I mean it to mean." It doesn't mean what it means in the dictionary. Let's take it to its extreme. Now you have freedom of speech, and you can say, "Well, speech is also expression." So speech means expression. It means you can do anything you want, anywhere, and any time you want. When does speech stop being speech? If we interpret speech means expression, then expression is action, and therefore the Ku Klux Klan is quite legal, isn't it? So is sedition, so is treason. So why not assassination? Oh, because there you hurt somebody else. Is that the only line between truth and falsehood? You can do, say, behave in any way so long as it doesn't injure somebody else physically. That brings us down to the very lowest dimension. That's lower than primitive tribes. Primitive tribes operated at a much higher level of moral integrity and social responsibility than whether or not your behavior is going to cause an actual physical energy.

#4: Contract the expertise of a very successful private enterprise to conduct vital operations.

An advisory council identifies this trend. By calibrating levels of consciousness, you can calibrate the energy of these various philosophies. The consequence of the perpetrators and supporters of relativism linking up with fascist theocracies in the far right are sufficient to destroy this civilization we call America.

Now calibrate that. It's the combination of those two, by means of iteration, nonlinear dynamics. One principle is sensitive dependence on initial conditions. If you have a defect in the 26th decimal point, which occurred in one of the most famous computers of recent times, you might say, "Oh, well, the twenty-sixth decimal point, so what." But by iteration, meaning by pushing that key tens of millions of times, you can bring down an entire building. The combination of those two together, I'll tell you as a self-appointed member of the advisory council, is sufficient to bring down our society. Before they become epidemic, the council would spot this. I think it's very neat from observation to have our calibrations to utilize private enterprise to conduct vital operations in business.

#5: Utilize an accurate, sophisticated intelligence capability, using consciousness calibration techniques to tell us what in the world is actually going on.

Let's look at the intelligence operations traditionally. If you operated a private big corporation, and you didn't know what your competition was up to, you'd soon be bankrupt. The calibrated level of integrity of our intelligence operations, before Pearl Harbor, 9/11, and so on, was a complete and total failure.

An advisory council, which has nothing to gain or nothing to lose, would say, "You've got to have some expert diagnosis. You don't just go and operate based on a guess or political viewpoint." It's like having the family join in on the operation. Now we're all going to vote. Can you imagine having a family looking over your shoulder while you're doing brain surgery? Not on my watch, I'll tell you.

With an advisory council and calibration techniques, we would have a much better grasp on these issues and better strategies to deal with them.

#6: Develop an international diplomacy based on precise, specific information obtainable by the techniques that we describe in this book and in this series of lectures.

International diplomacy. What is the country's nuclear intention? What is their nuclear capability? That's not up to politicians to guess about. Our survival depends on knowing what is the truth and the facts.

That's not a time for politics. You see, the advisory council is *beyond* politics. They're not interested in politics, except as an expression of that which is supportive and beneficial to the country and to the world in general. As I've mentioned in some of my lectures, I've been embarrassed by the way some representatives of America have behaved toward leaders of other countries. I can remember a TV interviewer interviewing the president of China. The president of China is president of the biggest country in the entire world, and this interviewer is going on about how China should look at this policy and adopt that policy. The president of China handled him very well, but I thought the interviewer was disrespectful, insulting, and showed a lack of sensitivity. An advisory council would advise against presenting yourself abrasively to other leaders of the world.

#7: Use trade alliances rather than power politics to facilitate and benefit our relationships with other countries.

Below 200, the only interest a country has is, "What's in it for us?" Well, one thing that's in it for us, we can see China, despite its supposedly a theoretical economic threat to the US, was a possible, very severe enemy. And even now some people would like to inflame it so that they could be. Why would they be? Their whole economy, the success of their economy, is based on their trade with the US. I think businesses like Walmart are doing more to prevent war with China probably than all the diplomats put together in the world.

International trade agreements are one way to preclude war, not just by buying out other countries. I don't believe in bribing them. If the US provides grants to foreign countries that hate them and those countries use the money to build missiles to destroy the US, the advisory council would say, "That's ridiculous." No, you have to make considerations intrinsic, that the trade then is dependent on certain factors. And these factors then ensure your security. You don't need ballistic missiles, unless you get a maniac as head of state because the maniac will kill his own population. Saddam called all his people dogs. Hitler said, "Burn down Paris. Burn down Germany. They deserve to die because they lost the war." Well, by the time they surface to the degree that even the most unconscious person can recognize who they are, it's too late.

So the advice is you diagnose cancer early in the game. You don't wait until it's metastasized to all the vital organs of the body. As a physician, I'm very interested in using this technique for early diagnosis to prevent the disease of mankind called death and destruction, starvation, and horrors of war.

What does it cost to do this? Nothing. Right now, it would take us about two seconds. We can reconfirm the positions of every country in the world—their nuclear capacity, their intention, et cetera, the level of their leaders—in five minutes flat. We would know in five minutes, more than all the collective diplomacy and intelligence operations in the whole world know right now. So you see why telling truth from falsehood is so mind-boggling. In one second, we can find out things that the international intelligence community is unable to discover. And even what they do discover is only a possibility or a probability, and the information may turn out to be false later on.

I'm interested in using muscle testing as a physician, for the benefit of society, for the prevention of war and in service of wisdom, because wisdom is truth and it's the service to God, to be of service to God. It's a selfless service, to utilize one's talents, one's abilities, one's energy, one's years of life to be of service to all of humanity as an expression of love, devotional non-duality. They call it devotion.

To close this section, Dr. Hawkins offers a prayer for readers to connect with the source of all existence, infinite silence, and to experience a feeling of being centered and grateful.

• • •

DEVOTIONAL NON-DUALITY PRAYER

"And therefore, I thought that which is the voice of God is silence, that we sink into the voice of God. We sink into the silence, which is indicative of divine presence. Behind the thought, behind the thinkingness is an infinite silence. And the infinite silence is the source of all existence. And between the thoughts, under the thoughts is the profound silence. And all we have to do is to become aware of that silence. All we have to do is become aware of that silence by realizing it's there.

"Behind all the sound of the universe, the silence is forever there. Behind the sounds in the woods, the woods are silent. The sound of the bird doesn't have anything to do with the silence. You see, the silence is maintained even though there's sound above it. But the only reason you can hear the sound is because it's against the background of silence. The silence is there right in the middle of sound.

"Focus on the silence, which is ever present, in the middle of cacophony and catastrophe, as the bullets are flying around and the planes are crashing and all hell's breaking loose, and there's nothing but the infinite silence. Identify with that silence and just maintain the awareness. Go about your daily life and do everything that you need to do, and at all times still be aware of the presence of the silence.

"That gives you a centering. A centering kind of prayerfulness is you're always aware of the silence, which is the infinite context. The reality of the presence of God is an infinite silence. And then that which you hold in mind in that silence tends to manifest, not as a result of causation but potentiality manifesting.

"And we thank thee, oh Lord, for thy divine presence as the infinite silence out of which arises our existence. Amen.

"And we finish with the same that we started, *Gloria in Excelsis Deo*. We thank thee, oh Lord, for thy divine presence. You are my gift. You're my gift from God. Thank you, God."

BONUS MATERIAL

The Most Valuable Qualities for a Spiritual Seeker

In this special bonus chapter, we share one of the last lectures that Dr. Hawkins delivered, which focuses on the most valuable qualities for a spiritual seeker.

We start with the certainty, knowing. Just know that if you're spiritually oriented, you will make progress. Start, therefore, with a feeling of security. Instead of insecurity or self-doubt, know that anybody who wants to evolve spiritually will receive the necessary assistance. Success is *guaranteed*. Get rid of self-doubt, any idea that you're not worth it, or that you're not capable of it, or that it's not the right time in your life. It's always the right time in your life. Accept without reservation that you are worthy of the quest. Be resolved to totally surrender to the truth about God. Surrender to the truth about God, and trust that your spiritual evolution is aligned with God's will for you. So always start with a feeling of security instead of self-doubt. The living proof of God's love and will for you is the gift of your own existence. The fact that you are, is the best evidence there is of God's love and will for you.

Here are the other valuable qualities for a spiritual seeker:

- **Do not compare yourself with others regarding holiness, merit, goodness, deservingness, sinlessness.** Do not compare yourself to others. What others are is irrelevant. What's important is what you are. Realize these are all human notions you have about being better. And God is not limited by human notions.

- **Accept that the concept of the "fear of God" is ignorance. God is peace and love, and nothing else.** There are lots of people who talk about the fear of God and use God as a threat. God is nothing but love and peace, and nothing else. People think that they're being punished by God, and that's not the case. What they're being punished by is their lack of alignment with divinity.

- **Realize that the depiction of God as a "judge" is a delusion, an ego fixation arising out of guilt. Realize that God is not a parent.** What God becomes in most people's minds is a parent who rewards you and loves you if you're good, and punishes you if you're bad. That's nothing but a parent. Realize that God is something greater than a parent.

- **Avoid negativity (calibrated levels below 200) and follow the goal to reach unconditional love (calibration level 540 and over).** What Jesus Christ wanted us to reach was unconditional love. Christ knew that once the level of unconditional love was reached, the soul's destiny was certain and the soul was safe. This is essentially the same teaching as the other great world religions, such as Judaism, Islam, and Buddhism. Sometimes spiritual seekers will become confused and wonder if they are following the right teacher or reading the right books. What you need to do is see that the essence of all of them is almost identical. The essence, not the surface of it, but the essence is almost identical.

• **Realize that salvation and enlightenment are somewhat different goals.** Salvation is concerned with yes or no. Enlightenment is concerned with becoming something beyond that which you have been. Salvation requires purification of the ego. Enlightenment is concerned with letting it go and eliminating the ego. The goal of enlightenment is somewhat more demanding than simply being a good person. Enlightenment is something other than good personhood. It's advancing one's level of consciousness in the nonlinear realms.

• **Clarify that it is not a personal you who is seeking enlightenment, but rather a quality of consciousness itself that is the motivator.** So, you like to think of *I am this* or *I am that.* And actually, it's merely consciousness itself, being what it is. Spiritual inspiration and dedication carry forth the work within yourself. Everybody has spiritual momentum.

• **Comfort replaces insecurity when one realizes that the most important goal has already been accomplished.** The goal is to be on the path.

• **Spiritual love, spiritual development is not an accomplishment, but a way of life.** It is an orientation that brings its own rewards. And what is important is the direction of one's own motives in life. There's no value in keeping the scorecard on yourself, the scorecard marking, "How far have I come?" or "How far do other people think I have come?" The only one you have to answer to is yourself. And the motivation to seek God is God. Nobody seeks God, except under the influence of divinity, because man left to his own device will never think of it.

- **Appreciate that every step forward brings benefits to everyone.** So, as you advance spiritually, it brings a value to everyone, to every human being. Because of the collective consciousness, every single person who improves helps to elevate the level of consciousness. And as that elevates, the incidence of war, suffering, ignorance, savaging, and disease diminish. When you advance yourself, you're helping everybody appreciate that every step forward benefits everyone. One's spiritual dedication and work is a gift to life and the love of mankind. It's nice to know that what you think you're doing only for yourself is actually benefiting everyone around you. To be kind to just one living being benefits everyone.

- **There is no timetable or prescribed route to God.** Although each person's route is unique, the terrain to be covered is relatively common to all. Whatever torments you go through in trying to perfect yourself, overcome sinfulness and selfishness, et cetera, realize that this is common to all of mankind. People troop into church Sunday mornings, everybody working on the same problem (how to be less selfish, how to be more giving, how to be more loving, et cetera).

- **The work is to surmount and transcend the common human failings that are inherent in the structure of the human ego.** Whatever defects you have are not just personal—they're not just yours. They are the problem of the human ego itself. And the problem is one of evolution that mankind at this point has evolved only to a certain point. One would like to think they are personal. However, the ego itself is not personal. People would like to think, *Oh, me and my progress, or me and my sins, or me and my difficulties*. And what you're talking about is not your personal self. The problem is that of the ego itself. And so, you stop taking the ego personally. When we realize it's really a collective problem that you share with all of mankind, that makes you feel a little less guilty. It's not the personal *I*, it's the human ego, which comes out of the structure of the brain itself, plus the human experience of life on this planet. We want to surmount and transcend the common human failings, they're inherent in the structure of the human ego. The human ego, not *your* ego, but the *human* ego. So you say, well, that is characteristic of the human ego.

- **The ego was inherited along with becoming a human being.** The ego is a product of the brain and the function of the brain. And details differ based on past karma of how this expresses itself. The ego is one thing, the brain function is another, and then you add to it past karma. Now, karma is not that well known in the Western world, but once you grab on to karma, you'll find that it's a very handy tool.

- **Intense prayer augments dedication and inspiration and facilitates progress.** We give loving service to all those who are around us, intense dedication, prayer, and an appeal to God: "Dear God, please help me in this endeavor." You call upon all the good karma you can think of, all the people you've been nice to, all the money you've put into the collection plate at church, all the old ladies you helped cross the street, all the starving little doggies that you gave something to eat.

- **The grace of God is available to everyone.** That's the most encouraging one of all. When you ask God for help, God's grace is available to everyone. Historically, the grace of the sage is available to the committed spiritual seeker. The consciousness of a spiritual teacher, especially the sage, radiates forth into the world. The grace of the sage is transmitted by the actual physical presence of the consciousness of the teacher.

I wished it would go via the written page, but the laws of consciousness are that the power of the teacher transmits into the consciousness of the student. And therefore, unfortunately, one does have to be in the actual physical presence of the teacher at some point in one's spiritual evolution. Happily, there's enough power in the teachers that are available, because it accumulates over time. So, the spiritual power of the great teachers who once lived, but are no longer in the living body, is still available, because it's transmitted down from one sage to the consciousness level of the next. But there is a definite value to being in the physical presence of the consciousness of the teacher.

- **The strength of the ego can be quite formidable.** And without the assistance of the power of a higher spiritual being, the ego cannot of itself be transcended, though one indirect benefit one gets from being in the physical presence of the consciousness field of an enlightened teacher is that it diminishes the hold of the ego and increases your power to transcend it. This is because of your own intention. With a person who does not wish this to happen, it will not happen. You say, "I refuse to listen to this guy. I'm not going to pay attention—he is full of bunk." Then that is what it will be with you. And things will remain the same. Skepticism and doubt, therefore, are not of any great service. The strength of the ego can be formidable. And without the assistance of the power of higher spiritual beings, ego cannot of itself transcend itself.

Fortunately, the power of the consciousness of every great teacher or avatar who has ever lived still remains and is available. To focus on a teacher or their teachings by meditation makes the power of that teacher available to the seeker. So down through the centuries, the power of the consciousness of the great beings is now present and calibrates true. It is now available to every student and is their karmic right.

It is your right, by virtue of your declaration, to benefit from the consciousness of all the great teachers who have ever lived.

ABOUT THE AUTHOR

David R. Hawkins PhD (1927–2012) was director of the Institute for Spiritual Research Inc. and founder of the Path of Devotional Nonduality. He was renowned as a pioneering researcher in the field of consciousness as well as an author, lecturer, clinician, physician and scientist. He served as an advisor to Catholic, Protestant and Buddhist monasteries; appeared on major network television and radio programmes; and lectured widely at such places as Westminster Abbey, the Oxford Forum, the University of Notre Dame and Harvard University. His life was devoted to the upliftment of mankind until his death in 2012.

For more information on Dr Hawkins's work, visit veritaspub.com

Hay House Titles of Related Interest

YOU CAN HEAL YOUR LIFE, the movie,
starring Louise Hay & Friends
(available as an online streaming video)
www.hayhouse.com/louise-movie

THE SHIFT, the movie,
starring Dr Wayne W. Dyer
(available as an online streaming video)
www.hayhouse.com/the-shift-movie

***

BECOMING SUPERNATURAL: How Common People Are Doing the Uncommon, by Dr Joe Dispenza

BLISS BRAIN: The Neuroscience of Remodeling Your Brain for Resilience, Creativity, and Joy, by Dawson Church

MIND TO MATTER: The Astonishing Science of How Your Brain Creates Material Reality, by Dawson Church

THE SCIENCE OF SELF-EMPOWERMENT: Awakening the New Human Story, by Gregg Braden

All of the above are available at www.hayhouse.co.uk

• • •

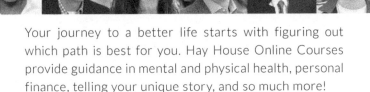

HAY HOUSE

Look within

Join the conversation about latest products,
events, exclusive offers and more.

 Hay House

 @HayHouseUK

 @hayhouseuk

We'd love to hear from you!